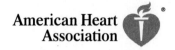

American Heart
Association

complete guide to
women's
heart
health

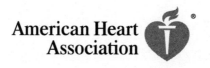

American Heart Association

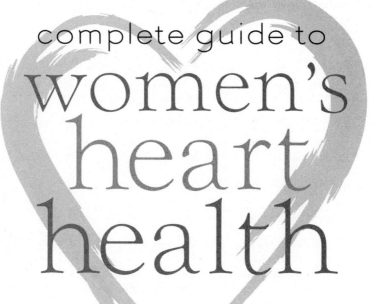

complete guide to

women's heart health

The **Go Red For Women®** Way
to Well-Being & Vitality

CLARKSON POTTER/PUBLISHERS
NEW YORK

Copyright © 2009 by the American Heart Association

Go Red and Go Red For Women® are trademarks of AHA.
The Red Dress Design is a trademark of U.S. DHHS.

No book, including this one, can ever replace the services of a doctor in providing information about your health. You should check with your doctor before using the information in this or any other health-related book.

Published in the United States by Clarkson Potter/Publishers, an imprint of the Crown Publishing Group, a division of Random House, Inc., New York.
www.crownpublishing.com
www.clarksonpotter.com

Clarkson Potter is a trademark and Potter with colophon is a registered trademark of Random House, Inc.

Your contributions to the American Heart Association support research that helps make publications like this possible.
For more information, call 1-800-AHA-USA1 (1-800-242-8721) or contact us online at www.americanheart.org.

Library of Congress Cataloging-in-Publication Data is available upon request.

ISBN 978-0-307-45060-9

Printed in the United States of America

Design by Stephanie Huntwork

1   3   5   7   9   10   8   6   4   2

First Edition

CONTENTS

PART THREE
health care for your heart

PART FOUR
resources

ACKNOWLEDGMENTS

American Heart Association Consumer Publications
Director: Linda S. Ball
Managing Editor: Deborah A. Renza
Senior Editor: Janice Roth Moss
Science Editor/Writer: Jacqueline F. Haigney
Assistant Editor: Roberta W. Sullivan

American Heart Association Science Advisors
Judy Bezanson, Science and Medicine Advisor
Dorothea Vafiadis, Science and Medicine Advisor
Nancy Haase, Statistics Consultant

YOUR HEART, OUR MISSION

BY ROSE MARIE ROBERTSON, M.D.

At the American Heart Association, we know heart health. We study it, we fund research on it, we write about it, and we invest our energies, time, and talents in it. Our mission is to build healthier lives, free of cardiovascular diseases and stroke. So, why is imparting information specifically about women's hearts so important to us? It's vital to share this information with you and other women because of the startling statistics that recent research has discovered concerning women's heart health. We know that right now, more than one in three women dies from cardiovascular disease. In fact, cardiovascular disease causes approximately one death every minute among women in the United States, and it claims more lives than any other cause of death. Additionally, more than 41 million American women are living with some form of this disease right now—that's about the entire current estimated population of New York, Michigan, and Ohio combined. That information alone is more than enough motivation for us to get this book into the homes of women across America.

The outlook is not completely hopeless, however. In fact, what we know for sure is that heart disease is actually largely preventable. The *American Heart Association Complete Guide to Women's Heart Health* will show you how your lifestyle choices, including what you eat and how much you exercise, can prevent or delay heart disease. What you need to do to keep your heart as healthy as possible is not rocket science, but it is science. Scientific studies tell us that eating a balanced diet and spending a little more than 1 percent of your time each week exercising moderately has a major impact not only on your heart's health but also on the vitality of your life.

What we *don't* know for sure are all the answers about how women's hearts are different from men's, as well as why heart disease and its treatments can affect women differently. Nevertheless, the American Heart Association is focused on advancing extensive research in this relatively new field of women's heart health. The future is encouraging, and the more knowledge we acquire, the more power we—as women ourselves—have to prevent heart disease.

If you've picked up this book, then you've already made an important first step in increasing your awareness of your own heart health. We encourage you to read the information inside for yourself and to share it with your mother, daughter, sisters, and girlfriends. We hope this book will empower you to start making good lifestyle choices *now* to reap the rewards of good heart health later. It's never too late—or too early—to take action to protect your heart.

Rose Marie Robertson is the Chief Science Officer of the American Heart Association/American Stroke Association.

american heart association
complete guide to women's heart health

EMPOWER YOURSELF
TO GO RED

BY NIECA GOLDBERG, M.D.

Red is the color of passion and strength. It is also the color of your body's lifeline—your cardiovascular system.

As a medical student I was fascinated by the way the heart pumps blood into a network of blood vessels throughout the body, and then later the blood returns to the lungs for oxygen and then gets pumped around again—the ultimate plumbing system. One day in anatomy class, when I was a student, I noticed that the artery I was studying felt stiff instead of rubbery and smooth. My professor informed me that the artery was atherosclerotic, that is, it was hardened because of cholesterol deposited in its walls. He also told me that it was a man's artery because heart disease was a man's disease.

I was reminded of this inaccurate and chauvinistic lesson some years ago when a publication from the American Heart Association reported that more women than men were dying from cardiovascular disease.

Today we know more. Although heart disease is still the leading killer of women, we have a lot more insight into prevention of heart disease in women. The American Heart Association launched the Go Red For Women® movement to educate women and their healthcare providers about the risks and symptoms of heart attacks.

But awareness is only half the battle. Information is power, but using that information is even more powerful. That's why as a cardiologist, the author of a successful women's health book, and the spokesperson for the Go Red For Women campaign, I speak to lots of women about heart health.

When I tell them that one in three women dies of cardiovascular disease, they look interested.

When I tell them that 64 percent of women who die suddenly of coronary heart disease had no previous symptoms and that many of those women had at least one risk factor that could have been treated, their jaws drop.

When I tell them that making healthy changes in their lives could reduce their risk for heart disease by as much as 80 percent, they look at me in disbelief.

But it's all true, and it's important information to act on.

Sometimes statistics like these are enough to motivate you to make changes in your life, like starting an exercise program, eating a healthier diet, or quitting smoking. But most of us have trouble getting started and sticking with a program because we have busy lives, including working and caring for children and sick parents. Who has the time? How do you begin? All you need is to Go Red. Adopt a way of life that will protect your lifeline—and you can begin by turning the pages of this book.

Nieca Goldberg is Clinical Associate Professor of Medicine of the New York University School of Medicine and spokesperson for the American Heart Association's Go Red For Women campaign.

Go Red For Women is the American Heart Association's national movement to increase women's awareness of their risk for heart disease, their number one killer, and to help them make the right choices to reduce their risks. The movement connects women with their own heart health and compels them to choose heart-healthy habits and supports the cause as they communicate with others about the choice to beat heart disease. For more information on Go Red For Women, visit GoRedForWomen.org.

american heart association
complete guide to women's heart health

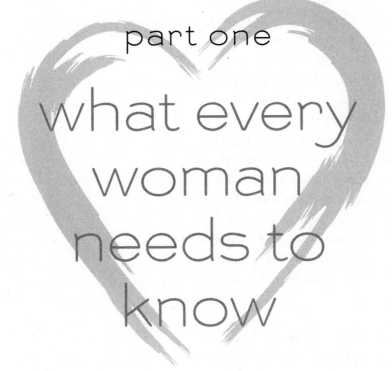

part one

what every
woman
needs to
know

CHAPTER I

your heart's health is in your hands

One in every three women dies of cardiovascular disease . . . but you don't have to be the one.

Cardiovascular disease is the greatest health risk for women. It causes more deaths than *all* forms of cancer combined! The good news is that although these grim statistics exist today, they don't have to— because **heart disease is largely preventable!**

Women today can benefit from the huge advances made by medical research. So much more is known and understood about prevention and the incredible importance of a heart-healthy lifestyle than was the case even 20 years ago. Statistics show that if a woman reaches her 50s without developing the major risk factors for heart disease, she will face only an 8 percent lifetime risk of developing cardiovascular disease—as opposed to a 50 percent risk if she develops two or more risk factors. Young women today—if they choose a heart-healthy lifestyle—may live their entire lives without getting heart disease!

Our deepened understanding of the long-term impact of the food and activity choices we make every day is an enormous breakthrough. Today's young women can benefit from the lifesaving information their mothers and grandmothers didn't have. You can protect yourself against heart disease for a lifetime. The science of prevention is so powerful—and so simple.

It's never too early to make your heart's health a priority. The earlier you start, the greater the benefit. A lifetime without heart disease is quite a payoff for eating your vegetables and exercising regularly.

Because heart disease is progressive and starts early in life and slowly escalates, older women also benefit from a healthy lifestyle. Controlling risk factors, eating right, being active, and working closely with your doctor can bring additional vitality and energy to your life.

With so much at stake, why doesn't every woman have a heart-healthy lifestyle? Because there are so many myths and misconceptions about heart disease, many women just don't understand they're at risk.

myth #1: heart disease only happens to men

Wrong. Cardiovascular disease, which includes coronary artery disease and stroke, is the leading cause of death for both men *and women.*

Heart disease in men has been well researched, and most men are aware it could happen to them, especially by the time they reach their 40s. But women are at risk too. This myth that women don't suffer from heart disease has persisted, in part, because women tend to have heart attacks about 10 years later than men do, in their mid- to late 50s. By the time women reach that age range, they also may have coexisting medical conditions that complicate the diagnosis.

Women's hearts are biologically different from men's—as can be their symptoms of heart disease and heart attack. In fact, the classic Hollywood heart attack—a man clutches his chest in extreme pain and falls to the ground—is not consistent with the reality of many heart attacks in either men or women.

Women's symptoms can be less dramatic but no less deadly. In women, heart attacks may manifest themselves as back pain, indigestion, breathlessness, weakness, dizziness, and a general feeling of malaise or "just not feeling well," as well as pain in the chest, the arm, and the jaw—or any combination of these symptoms. (For more information on the warning signs of heart attack, see Appendix E.)

The many ways these symptoms can vary have caused confusion for women and for their doctors, at times even leading to misdiagnosis or nondiagnosis of heart attack and heart disease. The vague nature of her symptoms can often cause a woman to delay seeking medical help—and may make her condition more difficult to diagnose after she has gone to the doctor or the emergency room. These delays may be the reason heart attacks are deadlier for women than for men.

Gender-specific research and improved practices throughout the medical community have led to gains in fighting cardiovascular disease, but women and their healthcare providers need to be vigilant about symptoms that could signal developing heart disease or a heart attack and then take action immediately.

myth #2: heart disease is just part of getting old

Wrong. Hearts do age, just as hair turns gray, but heart disease isn't an inevitable part of aging.

Older women often do develop heart disease because of the risk factors that started accumulating in their youth. High cholesterol, high blood pressure, obesity, diabetes, and other risk factors build and compound with age.

The plaque narrowing a 50-something woman's arteries probably started building up when she was in her 20s. High blood pressure in her 60s may have started with slightly elevated readings in her 30s.

Many of the conditions that escalate and compound to become **heart disease can be prevented by making good lifestyle choices**, especially eating a healthy diet, being physically active on a regular basis, and not smoking.

And if you are diagnosed with heart disease or have a history of heart disease in your family, don't give up! Your life isn't over. Medicine has made huge advances in treating heart disease. You can still benefit from a heart-healthy lifestyle; eating well and exercising regularly may slow the progression of your heart disease. Follow your doctor's directions, take all medications exactly as prescribed, and choose a healthy lifestyle.

myth #3: there's nothing i can do

Wrong again. Because many of the risk factors that lead to heart disease are lifestyle related, you can make an enormous difference in your health by making good choices every day. Stay away from cigarette smoke. Have the fish instead of the burger. Pick the baked chicken instead of the fried. Take the stairs instead of the elevator.

The simple healthy choices you make daily will compound, and you'll be healthier overall just as consistently making unhealthy choices will add up over the years and may show up as risk factors for heart disease.

The most important thing you can do is to accept that you're at risk and then act on that knowledge:

- **Be smart about your lifestyle.**

- **Be vigilant about changes in your body and its condition.**

- **Be an active partner with your doctor**—make sure you ask questions, tell him or her everything, and understand what your test results mean.

Although the medical treatment of heart disease is constantly improving, *prevention* is truly the "magic bullet" for this vital women's health issue. Heart disease develops gradually and progresses steadily.

You can gradually but steadily add heart-healthy habits to your lifestyle. You may think that doing the things that are good for your health on a regular basis—shopping for fruits and vegetables, cooking heart-healthy meals, developing a sustainable exercise program—seems like work. Well, it is work. It's the work of creating a healthy lifestyle, and that won't happen by chance.

The road to a heart-healthy lifestyle really is traveled one step at a time, one meal at a time, one day at a time. Not very dramatic, perhaps. Not nearly as alluring as the claims for "super" foods or "miracle" drugs or "power" exercises. But the dramatic reward you are working toward—a longer, healthier life—really does begin with your very next choice.

A Special Message for Women of Color

As a cardiologist, a researcher, and a woman, I want to give you a special warning: if you're a woman of color, you are at great risk for heart disease and heart attack. In fact, you are twice as likely to develop heart disease or have a heart attack as a Caucasian woman.

Many people think that heart disease is something that happens to men; the truth is that **women of black ancestry** (African American and Caribbean American) **and Hispanic women are at the highest risk for heart disease.**

Why are we women of color at increased risk for the number one killer of women? Race and genetics do play a role, but just as important is the fact that black and Hispanic women are more likely to have high blood pressure, to smoke, and to be physically inactive—all major risk factors for heart disease.

- Almost half of African American women and about one-third of Hispanic woman have high blood pressure.

- Almost three-quarters of both African American and Hispanic women in the United States are overweight or obese.

The finding that African American and Hispanic women have as much as a 69 percent higher risk of heart disease than Caucasian women is scary, but the solution to this problem isn't. Many women who have developed heart disease or had a heart attack might have been able to protect themselves by making lifestyle changes such as eating better, getting more exercise, and controlling other risk factors. It's not as hard as you might think to embrace a healthy lifestyle, but it does take planning and commitment. And the first step is being aware that as a woman of color you are at risk—increased risk.

You don't have to be a statistic.

JENNIFER H. MIERES, M.D.
Associate Professor of Medicine, New York University School of Medicine

CHAPTER 2

the heart of the matter: why your heart is so important

Your heart is the most vital organ in your body. From the minute you are born, your heart has the job of pumping blood throughout your body to deliver life-sustaining oxygen and nutrients to every cell. Each cell in the human body requires a constant supply of oxygen to create the energy it uses to stay alive. Since it takes only a few minutes without oxygen for a cell to die, **every heartbeat is important.** Any change that affects the ability of your heart to carry out its all-important mission will equally affect the quality of your overall health.

Given how crucial your heart is to your overall well-being, it makes sense to **do as much as you can to protect this precious organ and its supporting circulatory system throughout your life,** not just when you are older. Maintaining your health at a cellular level will help to prevent damage that can lead to disease and death.

how your heart works

The heart is a four-chambered muscular pump a little larger than your fist. Each day, it empties and refills about 100,000 times in a sequence of highly organized contractions. Pumping at an average rate of 72 beats per minute, your heart keeps your blood moving with sufficient pressure to provide a constant supply of nutrients to all your cells, from the top of your brain to the tips of your toes—and back again. A lot has to happen in one heartbeat to maintain this remarkable pumping power. To function effectively, your heart depends on four components:

- four heart chambers made of muscle tissue

- four heart valves

- an anatomic (natural) pacemaker and conduction system to initiate and deliver the electrical stimulus for each contraction

- the circulatory network of arteries and veins that bring blood into the heart, send it out to the lungs, and finally move it on to the rest of the body

The Heart Itself

The heart is divided into right and left sides, separated by a wall called the septum. Each side has an upper chamber, the **atrium,** and a lower chamber, the **ventricle.** The atria receive blood and move it on to the ventricles. The left ventricle is the largest, most powerful, and hardest working of the heart's chambers because it has to be able to pump forcefully enough to move blood through the body against the resistance of gravity. The entire heart is surrounded by the **pericardium,** a protective membrane that holds the heart in place yet allows it to move during its cycle of contractions.

A specialized group of cells in the heart muscle (or myocardium) produces electrical impulses that cause the heart chambers to contract in sequence. Located in the right atrium, the sinoatrial node acts as the heart's natural pacemaker, coordinating the signals to tell the upper chambers, the atria, to contract simultaneously. There is a slight pause to give the ventricles time to fill with blood, and then these lower chambers contract, also at the same time. This creates the two-tone "lub-dub, lub-dub" sound of the heartbeat.

Valves in the Heart

Between the chambers are valves that open and close to keep the blood moving in one direction only. Between the right atrium and ventricle is

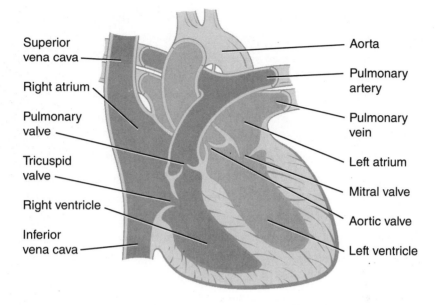

Superior vena cava

Right atrium

Pulmonary valve

Tricuspid valve

Right ventricle

Inferior vena cava

Aorta

Pulmonary artery

Pulmonary vein

Left atrium

Mitral valve

Aortic valve

Left ventricle

the **tricuspid valve,** which allows blood to move into the right ventricle. Leading from the right ventricle, the **pulmonary valve** controls the flow of blood on its way to the lungs. Between the left atrium and left ventricle is the **mitral valve.** From the left ventricle, the blood flows through the **aortic valve** to the aorta and on to the coronary arteries and the rest of the body.

The Circulatory System

Arteries and veins circulate blood from the heart to other parts of the body and back again. Blood that has been circulated enters the right side of the heart through veins coming from the upper body (superior vena cava) and the lower body (inferior vena cava). The blood is pumped through the right side of the heart to the pulmonary artery, which sends it to the lungs to pick up oxygen and release the waste product carbon dioxide. The blood returns via the pulmonary veins to the left atrium. The blood then moves to the left ventricle, which pumps it to the aorta, the major artery that sends the now oxygen-rich blood on to do its job of feeding the body's cells. An elaborate network of 20 major arteries feeds smaller arteries, the **arterioles,** that branch off into the even smaller **capillaries,** with walls thin enough to allow the exchange of oxygen and nutrients for carbon dioxide and other waste products in the body's cells. (Some capillaries are so thin only a single blood cell can travel through at a time.) The blood then returns to the heart through **venules** that widen to become **veins,** then even larger veins. A series of valves in the large veins keep the blood traveling up toward the heart.

The circulatory system is an important contributor in regulating blood flow and completing the heart's job of providing vital oxygen and nutrients to your entire body. When you are exercising, for example, your muscle cells need energy, and therefore more oxygen. The heart responds by beating harder and faster to pump a greater volume of oxygen-rich blood. At the same time, your arteries expand to move the blood more quickly. When you stop exercising and cool down, the heart slows and the arteries return to their original diameter. Both arteries and arterioles help regulate blood pressure by widening and narrowing in response to signals from nerve fibers located in the blood vessel walls. The nerve fibers can be regulated by electrical messages from the nervous system as well as signals from other sources.

The Heartbeat Cycle: Movement of Blood Through the Heart

A subtle combination of pressure and flow keeps blood moving in distinct phases. Between heartbeats, oxygen-depleted blood collects in the right atrium. At the same time, oxygenated blood from the lungs flows into the left atrium. Reacting to the electrical signal from the sinoatrial node, both right and left atria contract simultaneously, forcing blood from the atria through the tricuspid and mitral valves, respectively, into the ventricles. Because of the pressure from the blood that has filled the ventricles, the tricuspid and mitral valves shut. The filling of the heart chambers is called the **diastolic phase.** As the electrical signal from the sinoatrial node travels across the heart, the atria relax and the right and left ventricles contract vigorously, the pulmonary and aortic valves open, and blood is propelled into the lungs from the right ventricle and to the aorta from the left ventricle. This contraction of the heart is called the **systolic phase.** As the ventricles relax, the pressure of the blood that has moved through and forward pushes back against the valves to close them. Since the pressure in the ventricles is reduced, the atrial valves can open again, so the entire sequence can start again.

This cycle repeats itself about 70 times every minute when you are at rest, moving blood through the circulatory system at a rate of about 100 gallons every hour. How much blood is pumped depends on how many times your heart beats, as well as the volume of blood pumped by the ventricles. The efficiency of the heart valves and the balance of pressure in the chambers keep the blood moving, and in only one direction:

right atrium → right ventricle → lungs for oxygen → left atrium →
left ventricle → aorta

From the aorta it moves to the coronary arteries located on the outer surface of the heart, and on throughout the circulatory system.

Like other organs, the heart also needs oxygen and nutrients, so it feeds itself first by sending about 4 to 5 percent of the oxygen-rich blood in the aorta through the **coronary arteries.** The coronary arteries surround the heart like a crown (hence the term "coronary") and branch into the heart muscle to supply it with oxygen-rich blood. Branching from the aorta, the left main coronary artery and the right coronary artery divide again into a network of smaller vessels that deliver blood to the different parts of the heart's muscle and electrical system. Like the larger circulatory system, the heart also has a network of veins that returns oxygen-poor blood to the right atrium, where it is re-circulated with the other blood returning from the body.

The complex interplay of these components of the cardiovascular system and their effective interaction with the other systems in your body are crucial in keeping you healthy and vigorous. When one or more of these components is compromised, your health and your body's ability to function are negatively affected in many ways, even if those effects are not immediately obvious to you.

risk factors for heart disease

To adapt to changes in your level of activity and emotional state, your brain and nervous system send signals to regulate the functions of your cardiovascular system. Your heart and circulatory system in turn must constantly regulate blood flow to meet the needs of your body, both at rest and during physical activity. **Over time, the combined influences of genetic predisposition and unhealthy lifestyle choices create the risk factors that threaten the efficiency of this intricate network.** These risk factors can lead to coronary artery disease and other conditions that further compromise the heart and circulatory system. (See Chapter 10 for an explanation of some of these common conditions.) The more you understand how to reduce your risk factors, the more you can do to protect your remarkable heart and its supporting systems.

What Is a Risk Factor?

Risk factors are conditions or behaviors that over time contribute to the development of coronary artery disease and other types of cardiovascular disease such as peripheral vascular disease, high blood pressure, and heart failure. Importantly, managing your risk factors through healthy lifestyle choices will positively impact your heart and blood vessels. Over time, however, damage to your heart and blood vessels can lead to emergency medical conditions such as heart attack or stroke. Both of these medical emergencies can lead to a lack of blood flow that restricts the delivery of oxygen to the cells in your body, specifically the heart or the brain.

In a medical context, the term **major risk factors** refers to those variables that research has shown significantly increase your chance of developing cardiovascular disease. The American Heart Association has designated smoking, physical inactivity, increasing age, genetic predisposition from family history or race, high blood pressure, high blood cholesterol levels, obesity, and diabetes as major risk factors. **Contributing risk factors** such as stress and excessive alcohol use are associated with an increased risk of cardiovascular disease, but a direct link hasn't been clearly demonstrated.

In practical terms, the greater the extent of each risk factor and the more risk factors you have, the greater the likelihood that you will develop heart disease. Having a risk factor, however, does not always lead to heart disease and, conversely, not having a risk factor does not mean that you will not develop heart disease.

Some risk factors can't be changed. You are going to get older, of course, and your heart ages with you. Research on the influence of genetics is showing that people may inherit a predisposition to certain risk factors. Likewise, race and gender influence your risk, and as more research is conducted on women and ethnic groups, we are learning more about how to translate study results into practical applications for managing different risks in different populations.

Many of the most damaging risk factors, however, are things that you *can* control. Smoking, being physically inactive, and eating many high-calorie foods are choices, not givens. Likewise, with a healthy lifestyle, you may be able to prevent or delay the major risk factors of high blood pressure, high blood cholesterol, and type 2 diabetes. If you already have any of these conditions, you can reduce the damage they do by eating well, being physically active, and taking medication as needed.

Risk Factors Beyond Your Control

INCREASING AGE
It is true that as you get older, the heart muscle and circulatory system undergo changes in structure and function that are considered a normal part of aging. These changes in themselves do not cause heart disease, however. Rather, as you get older you are more likely to develop risk factors that contribute to the accumulation of plaque in your arteries, as well as conditions that affect blood flow, such as high blood pressure.

GENETIC PREDISPOSITION
Family history
Research into the relationship between genetics and disease suggests that a number of genes are associated with a tendency to develop heart disease, stroke, and high blood pressure. Remember, however, that the impact of each individual gene on an individual woman is not yet fully

understood. If you have a congenital heart defect, for example, you are slightly more likely to have a baby with a congenital heart defect, and scientists are working to identify the associated genes. **If your parents or grandparents have or had heart disease, you are probably more likely to develop it, too.** Your risk is increased if a close blood relative had symptoms at an early age (for example, a heart attack or stroke before age 55 for male relatives or age 65 for female relatives). Most people with a strong family history of heart disease have one or more other risk factors as well, so it's even more important to treat and control them and reduce your risk by adopting a healthy lifestyle. If you know your family has a recurring history of risk factors such as high blood pressure, high LDL cholesterol, low HDL cholesterol, or diabetes, you can be better prepared to take the necessary steps to avoid developing similar problems.

Learn as much as you can about the medical histories of your parents, grandparents, and other blood relatives, such as aunts and uncles, on both sides of your family. (For a family history tree template, see Appendix D.) Has anyone in your immediate family suffered a heart attack or stroke? Do your relatives have major risk factors such as high blood pressure, high cholesterol, or diabetes? If so, you are predisposed to these conditions as well. **You may have to probe for relevant information for older female relatives, since heart disease was often overlooked in women in the past.** For example, if someone in your family remembers that your grandmother often complained about vacuuming or carrying groceries because they made her tired or out of breath, this could be an indicator that perhaps she had heart failure or another cardiovascular condition.

Ethnicity

Race can also be a risk factor. Although heart disease is the number one killer of *all* women of all ethnic backgrounds, the **major risk factors are more prevalent in African American and Hispanic women than in white women.** The prevalence of heart disease is also higher among some Native American, native Hawaiian, and Asian American populations. African Americans have a higher risk of developing high blood pressure, high cholesterol, and diabetes, which makes their risk of

american heart association
complete guide to women's heart health

heart disease and stroke greater. Smoking, physical inactivity, and being overweight or obese further increase that risk. Hispanic women also are at greater risk because of their higher rates of overweight/obesity, diabetes, and metabolic syndrome. If you know you are at risk because of your ethnicity or family history, be sure to do all you can to lessen your chances of developing heart disease.

If you are an African American woman, make it a priority to have your blood pressure checked regularly. Studies show that black women—even when very young—are much more susceptible to high blood pressure than white women. Not only is the disease more common among black women, but often it is more serious when it does develop.

Risk Factors You Can Prevent or Manage

HIGH BLOOD PRESSURE

Blood pressure is controlled by the network of arterioles, capillaries, and veins in your circulatory system. When these vessels constrict, the heart has to work harder to pump blood and deliver oxygen. The relationship of high blood pressure to cardiovascular disease is direct: the higher the blood pressure, the greater the risk.

Blood pressure is measured as both the pressure exerted against an artery wall when the heart contracts, called systolic pressure, and the pressure in the artery when the heart is at rest between beats, called diastolic pressure. Reported in millimeters of mercury (mmHg), these values are shown as systolic over diastolic pressure, so the readings are given as a fraction, for example, 120/80 mmHg or 120 over 80. Blood pressure varies from one part of the body to another, at different times of day, with different levels of anxiety or exertion, and even with body posture, but consistently higher-than-normal readings indicate a problem in the mechanism that regulates blood pressure. Called the silent killer, high blood pressure often has no symptoms, so the only way to identify it is to have your blood pressure checked regularly.

Blood pressure that measures over 140/90 mmHg on two separate occasions is classified as high, or **hypertension.** Normal blood pressure is defined as systolic pressure less than 120 mmHg and diastolic less than 80 mmHg. Slightly elevated blood pressure approaching unhealthy limits is called **prehypertension.**

BLOOD PRESSURE LEVEL	SYSTOLIC (mmHg)		DIASTOLIC (mmHg)
Normal	less than 120	and	less than 80
Prehypertension	120 to 139	or	80 to 89
Hypertension	140 or greater	or	90 or greater

Note: For adults 18 years or older. These levels apply only to people who are not taking medication for high blood pressure and who do not have a short-term serious illness.

How does high blood pressure increase the risk of heart disease? Over time, the constant force of added pressure causes artery walls to thicken and lose elasticity. The thickening narrows the space inside the artery, reducing blood flow and increasing the risk of a blood clot being trapped and stopping the flow completely. As the heart works harder to pump blood, it also grows larger, and the heavy workload eventually will take its toll by weakening the heart so it cannot pump effectively. Untreated high blood pressure significantly increases the risk of heart failure, heart attack, stroke, and kidney failure. According to the Framingham Heart Study (a cardiovascular study based in Framingham, Massachusetts, that examined more than 5,000 adults), when high blood pressure exists with smoking, high blood cholesterol levels, or diabetes, the risk of coronary heart disease or stroke increases even more.

Because **blood pressure is affected by many factors under your control,** your first line of defense is a healthy lifestyle that includes regular aerobic physical activity, such as brisk walking, and a diet low in sodium and saturated fat. Your diet should be high in vegetables and fruit, whole grains, and fat-free and low-fat dairy products. Quitting smoking, managing stress, and limiting alcohol to moderate amounts are also important to keep blood pressure low. When these strategies are not enough, you may need some form of medication, either a single drug or a combination. The options include diuretics, beta-blockers, calcium channel blockers, angiotensin-converting enzyme (ACE) inhibitors, and alpha-blockers.

UNHEALTHY LEVELS OF CHOLESTEROL
AND TRIGLYCERIDES

Cholesterol is one of several fatty substances called **lipids.** Your body needs cholesterol to form and strengthen cell walls and for other body functions, such as producing hormones and bile. Your blood carries cholesterol and other fats through your body in distinct particles called **lipoproteins.** (Because lipids, like other fats, do not mix with water, the body wraps them in protein to move them through the bloodstream.) Three types of lipoprotein make up the major part of your total blood cholesterol measurement: low-density lipoprotein (LDL), high-density lipoprotein (HDL), and very-low-density lipoprotein (VLDL).

Your liver produces the cholesterol in your blood. If your liver produces a high level of **LDL cholesterol** (the "bad" cholesterol), that excess contributes to a process called *atherosclerosis*. Atherosclerosis is a gradual buildup of fatty streaks that harden into plaque lining the arterial walls, increasing your risk of coronary heart disease and heart attack. These deposits of plaque narrow the arteries and reduce the flow of blood. If plaque cracks or ruptures, it triggers the formation of a blood clot. That clot can block blood flow where it is, or break off and travel to another part of the body to block flow elsewhere, causing a heart attack or stroke. This risk is why it's important to keep LDL cholesterol levels down. Conversely, a low level of **HDL cholesterol** (the "good" cholesterol) is also a risk factor for heart disease, especially in women. Because high-density lipoproteins appear to carry cholesterol away from existing plaque, higher levels of HDL cholesterol may protect against heart disease.

Triglycerides, another form of blood lipid and the most common type of fat in your body, are used for energy, unlike cholesterol. (The fats in food are also a form of triglyceride.) Whenever your body does not use all the calories you've eaten in a meal, the excess calories are stored as triglycerides and are carried in the blood by very-low-density lipoprotein. High levels of triglycerides usually accompany high LDL and low HDL cholesterol and other risk factors for disease and are linked with coronary heart disease. Although the exact mechanism is still unclear, triglycerides may contribute to atherosclerosis and thicken the blood, increasing the risk of arterial blockage and blood clots.

Work with your healthcare provider to determine your goal levels for blood cholesterol. What's right for you will depend on your current health situation and other risk factors, as well as your age and family history. In most cases, doctors' recommendations follow these general guidelines. Aim for:

✓ Total cholesterol of less than 200 mg/dL

✓ **LDL cholesterol less than 160 mg/dL if you have no heart disease or diabetes, with one or no other risk factors**

✓ **LDL cholesterol less than 130 mg/dL if you have no heart disease or diabetes, with two or more other risk factors**

✓ **LDL cholesterol less than 100 mg/dL if you have existing heart disease or diabetes** (Some high-risk patients may have a goal of less than 70 mg/dL.)

✓ **HDL cholesterol of 50 mg/dL or higher**

✓ **A triglyceride level of less than 150 mg/dL**

DIABETES

Diabetes, or diabetes mellitus, is a chronic disease that cannot be cured but can be successfully managed with proper care. If left untreated, it increases your risk for cardiovascular disease two to four times and can lead to serious long-term damage to your heart and kidneys. Even when glucose levels are under control, diabetes greatly increases your risk of heart disease and stroke. **The death rate for heart disease in adults with diabetes is about two to four times higher than in those without diabetes.** In fact, most women with diabetes die of some form of heart or blood vessel disease.

The hormone insulin controls the transfer of glucose from the bloodstream to the cells in the body. In the most common form of diabetes, type 2, either the pancreas does not produce enough insulin or the cells cannot use existing insulin. When the transfer of glucose breaks down, cells begin to starve and become damaged. Since the cells cannot take in glucose, the excess builds up in the blood. A simple blood test can identify a higher-than-normal level of blood glucose.

Insulin resistance occurs when the body can't use insulin efficiently. To compensate, the pancreas releases more and more insulin to try to keep blood sugar levels normal. Gradually, the insulin-producing cells in the pancreas become defective and decrease in number. As a result, blood glucose levels begin to rise, resulting in full-blown diabetes.

Diabetes is defined as a fasting blood glucose level of 126 mg/dL or more. **Prediabetes,** or impaired fasting glucose (IFG), is defined as a fasting blood glucose level between 100 and 125 mg/dL. Prediabetes is often present with other risk factors for heart disease in a condition known as metabolic syndrome.

The **metabolic syndrome** is closely associated with insulin resistance. The term refers to a combination of any three of the following risk factors: a waist measurement of 35 inches or greater for women; a triglyceride level of 150 mg/dL or higher; HDL cholesterol less than 50 mg/dL in women; systolic blood pressure of 130 mmHg or higher, or diastolic blood pressure of 85 mmHg or higher; and a fasting glucose reading of 100 mg/dL or higher. The combination of these risk factors is strongly associated with cardiovascular disease and other diseases related to plaque buildup in artery walls (for example, coronary artery disease, stroke, and peripheral artery disease) as well as type 2 diabetes.

Diabetes has a significant impact on women, because the disease can affect both mothers and their unborn children. Diabetes can cause difficulties during pregnancy such as a miscarriage or a baby born with birth defects. Gestational diabetes, a type of diabetes that arises during pregnancy, can increase the risk of developing diabetes after the baby is born. If you are diagnosed as having diabetes or insulin resistance, your doctor will prescribe changes in eating habits, weight control, a regular exercise program, and medication to keep your blood glucose levels in check. It's critical for women with diabetes to have regular checkups.

Risk Factors You Can Avoid or Control

SMOKING

Smoking is the number one preventable cause of premature death in the United States. There is no doubt that smoking tobacco products and constant exposure to secondhand smoke put you at greater risk for heart disease, stroke, and other illnesses. **A smoker's risk of dying from coronary heart disease is two to three times that of a nonsmoker's.** Smoking by itself raises the risk of coronary heart disease, but when you add smoking to other risk factors, the potent combination poses an even greater risk of disease. Smoking increases blood pressure, decreases capacity for exercise, and increases the tendency for blood to clot.

When you inhale smoke, you are also taking in chemicals such as nicotine and carbon monoxide. Nicotine causes arteries to constrict and become narrower, reducing blood flow and forcing the heart to work harder. This causes increased blood pressure and heart rate. At the same time, carbon monoxide binds to the hemoglobin in blood that normally carries oxygen from the lungs, reducing the amount of oxygen that reaches your body's cells. Smoking also promotes the accumulation of atherosclerosis, further reducing blood flow and narrowing arteries.

Studies show that on average, **women who smoke die more than 14 years earlier than those who do not smoke.** Smoking is an issue for the whole family: exposure to environmental tobacco smoke significantly increases the risk of health problems in women and children, including spontaneous abortions, fetal brain damage, low birth weight, sudden infant death syndrome, and mental retardation. And if you combine smoking with taking birth control pills, your risk of blood clotting and heart attack is greatly increased. So, **if you smoke, you must find a way to quit.** Although nicotine is addictive, many effective treatments are available to help you quit. Ask your healthcare provider to help you find a strategy that will work for you, including counseling, nicotine replacement, or other forms of therapy.

PHYSICAL INACTIVITY

Despite scientific evidence showing that being inactive increases the risk for heart disease, about 70 percent of all American women are sedentary and get no regular leisure-time physical activity. **The disease risk associated with physical inactivity is comparable to that for high blood cholesterol, high blood pressure, or smoking.** Inactive women are almost twice as likely as their more vigorous counterparts to develop coronary heart disease.

To put these numbers in perspective, **the risk of living an inactive life seems to be roughly equivalent to that of smoking a pack of cigarettes a day.** Some researchers have estimated that stepping up the pace of the American lifestyle from sedentary to active could reduce heart disease risk by one-third.

How does exercise reduce your risk? Like other muscles, your heart becomes stronger when it works hard on a regular basis. When it is conditioned through regular exercise, it beats more slowly but more effectively, so each beat pumps out more oxygen-rich blood. At rest, a well-conditioned heart delivers what's needed with less work. With exertion, a strong heart can work harder to deliver more oxygen-rich blood at a lower heart rate and lower blood pressure. As your heart is getting in condition, so are all the other muscles you exercise. They develop a greater number of capillaries (tiny blood vessels) and become more efficient at extracting the oxygen they need from your blood. Therefore, the same amount of movement or work will take less energy. In addition to increasing the efficiency of your cardiovascular system, physical activity can help control LDL and improve HDL cholesterol, fight diabetes and obesity, and lower blood pressure.

OVERWEIGHT AND OBESITY

As a result of recent lifestyle trends that tend to increase calorie intake and decrease physical activity, more than half the women in the United States are either overweight or obese. If you are one of them, you can dramatically reduce your risk of heart disease by reaching and maintaining a healthy weight. **Losing just 10 percent of your body weight will help lower your risk.**

How do extra pounds create problems for your health? To carry the extra weight, your body needs more energy, so your heart must work harder to provide more oxygen to your body's cells. Over time, this heavier workload causes the heart to enlarge and weaken. Extra weight also raises blood pressure: women who are obese are twice as likely to have high blood pressure as those at a healthy weight. Consistently taking in too many calories and eating a diet high in unhealthy fats increases blood levels of harmful LDL cholesterol and triglycerides while lowering helpful HDL cholesterol. Being overweight or obese also increases the likelihood of developing diabetes.

Research also has established a link between excess body fat—especially abdominal fat—and inflammation, which may also raise risk. Inflammation is a normal response to many physical states, including fever, injury, and infection, as well as to the progression of cardiovascular disease. The inflammatory process may damage the lining of arteries and/or cause arterial plaque to rupture, possibly triggering a heart attack.

Obesity is classified as a disease itself, yet it also is a risk factor for heart attack and heart disease, including coronary artery disease, congestive heart failure, cardiomyopathy (weakness of the heart muscle), and irregular heart rhythms. If you are obese and have more than two major risk factors, such as diabetes, high blood pressure, and high LDL cholesterol and triglycerides, the risk of heart disease and stroke is especially great.

Why are lower levels of drinking recommended for women than for men? Because women are at greater risk than men for developing alcohol-related problems. As a drink is consumed, the alcohol passes through the digestive tract and is dispersed in the water in the body. Since women are generally smaller overall than men, their bodies contain less water, pound for pound. The less water available, the less the alcohol can be diluted. Therefore, a woman's brain and other organs are exposed to more of the toxic byproducts that result when alcohol is broken down and eliminated by the body. Even when they drink less alcohol than men, women still suffer more physical damage.

EXCESSIVE ALCOHOL INTAKE

Drinking too much alcohol can raise blood pressure, increase risk of heart failure and stroke, and produce irregular heartbeats. Excessive alcohol use also can contribute to high triglycerides, breast cancer and other diseases, obesity, alcoholism, suicide, and accidents. Given these and other risks, the American Heart Association cautions women NOT to start drinking if they do not already drink alcohol. Research does show some evidence that *moderate* use of alcohol may protect your heart. What is considered moderate drinking? The American Heart Association recommends no more than one drink a day for women. One drink is defined as 1½ fluid ounces of 80-proof spirits (such as bourbon, Scotch, and vodka), 1 fluid ounce of 100-proof spirits, 4 fluid ounces of wine, or 12 fluid ounces of beer.

STRESS

Stress is an undeniable part of life. As the demands of modern life mount, so do the sleepless nights, headaches, stiff muscles, clenched teeth, irritability, and many other symptoms of chronic stress. Factoring in the everyday stresses of commuting, work-related travel, day care, marital issues, financial worries, and time pressure—it's no wonder that most women need to learn how to de-stress.

When you experience stress, your body undergoes physical changes called the *fight-or-flight response*. Reacting to triggers from your nervous system and the release of hormones (adrenaline, for example), your heart rate increases and your muscles tense so you will be better prepared to either fend off a threat or run away. Other changes that you may be less aware of include a rise in blood pressure, an increase in the clotting ability of your blood, constricted blood vessels, and a release of stored fat for quick energy. All these physical changes place an added burden on your heart and arteries as they must work harder to respond to the need for more oxygen-rich blood.

Everyone reacts in an individual way to life's stresses. An event that makes one woman's blood pressure soar may not even catch another's attention. Likewise, the physical reaction to stress varies greatly from woman to woman, as does each person's ability to manage her unique stresses. It's known that chronic stress can result in unhealthy lifestyle habits that increase the risk of heart disease. Smoking, drinking alcohol in excess, eating for comfort, rationalizing couch-potato behavior, and other self-defeating ways of coping don't deal with the source of the problem; they only mask the symptoms. For some women, physical reactions to stress may cause actual damage to the circulatory system, making them more vulnerable to plaque buildup and even heart attack.

Although the causal relationship between stress and heart disease has been difficult to establish, **most healthcare professionals consider ongoing stress a risk factor for heart disease and stroke.** Many of the reactions to stress, such as anxiety, back pain, tightness in the chest, and palpitations, are also signs of heart disease. If you experience these symptoms, talk to your doctor about the stresses in your life and your risk for cardiovascular issues. Even if you have no symptoms, you should take stress seriously as a health threat that you can learn to manage in healthy ways.

know the warning signs of heart attack

Even if you carefully manage your risk factors and do all you can to take care of your heart, it's wise to know the symptoms of heart attack. Although some women's heart attacks are sudden and intense—the "movie heart attack," where no one doubts what's happening—the fact is that **most heart attacks start slowly, with mild pain or discomfort.** As in men, chest pain or discomfort is the most common heart attack symptom in women. However, **women are more likely to experience some of the other common symptoms, particularly shortness of breath, nausea and/or vomiting, and back or jaw pain.** In addition, research suggests that indigestion and increasing fatigue may be experienced among some women having a heart attack.

Remember that not all warning signs occur with every heart attack. Often people affected aren't sure what's wrong and wait too long before getting help. **If you have one or more of the following signs, don't wait longer than 5 minutes before calling 9-1-1 for help.**

- **Chest discomfort.** Most heart attacks involve discomfort in the center of the chest that lasts more than a few minutes, or that goes away and comes back. The discomfort can feel like uncomfortable pressure, squeezing, fullness, or pain.

- **Discomfort in other areas of the upper body.** Symptoms can include pain or discomfort in one or both arms, the back, the neck, the jaw, or the stomach.

- **Shortness of breath.** This may occur with or without chest discomfort.

- **Other signs.** These may include breaking out in a cold sweat, nausea, or lightheadedness.

know the warning signs of stroke

A heart attack isn't the only dangerous manifestation of cardiovascular disease. Similar to a heart attack, a stroke can be considered a "brain attack." Stroke occurs when the flow of blood to the brain is obstructed or blocked by a clot located either in the arteries leading to the brain or in the brain, or by a blood vessel rupturing. When the obstruction or blockage happens, the affected part of the brain cannot get the oxygen and nutrients it needs and the cells start to die.

Because stroke happens so quickly, it is crucial to be familiar with the warning signs. Not all warning signs occur with every stroke.

- Sudden *numbness or weakness* of the face, arm, or leg, especially on one side of the body

- Sudden *confusion, trouble speaking,* or trouble understanding

- Sudden *trouble seeing* in one or both eyes

- Sudden *trouble walking, dizziness,* or *loss of balance* or coordination

- Sudden, severe *headache* with no known cause

If you or someone with you has one or more of these signs, don't delay! Immediately call 9-1-1 or, if needed, a separate emergency medical service (EMS) number, so an ambulance (ideally with advanced life support) can be sent. Also, check the time so you'll know when the first symptoms appeared. It's very important to **take immediate action.** If given within three hours of the start of symptoms, a clot-busting drug called tissue plasminogen activator (tPA) can reduce long-term disability for the most common type of stroke. tPA is the only FDA-approved medication for the treatment of stroke within three hours of symptom onset.

why is heart disease different in women

Although the basic anatomy of the heart is the same for women and men, there are important differences in the particulars, especially when it comes to heart disease. Not only are most women's hearts and arteries smaller than most men's, but **many women experience heart disease and heart attack differently than men.** Awareness of these differences has begun to filter through the medical community, as new studies have been focused specifically on women and heart disease. The Women's Health Initiative, Nurses' Health Study, and Women's Health Study are examples of the groundbreaking work that has helped challenge existing assumptions about diagnosis and treatment choices for women with heart disease.

To make reliable recommendations, medical researchers need time to review and compare study findings, follow up with further testing to verify conclusions, and extrapolate the implications for medical care. Clinicians also need time to understand the new knowledge and learn how to best apply it in their treatment of patients. The recent shift in how the medical community perceives heart disease in women is a good example of this process. Until 1986, when federal regulations were instituted to increase the inclusion of women in funded studies, the medical research on heart disease had been done predominantly on men. The findings of those studies were then generalized into the guidelines doctors used for clinical diagnosis and treatment of all patients. It was assumed that the guidelines would be equally effective in men and women, but that turned out not to be true. Because those guidelines were based on findings in men, heart disease in women who experienced different, or atypical, symptoms often went unrecognized or untreated. After years of treating women whose heart disease didn't seem to fit the conventional wisdom, however, many doctors and researchers began rethinking their approach.

In the late 1990s, researchers began to understand that the "classic" symptom of coronary artery disease or heart attack as experienced by men—severe pain in the center of the chest—may not always occur in women. Instead, **women may experience other types of symptoms,** such as fatigue, nausea or vomiting, and back, stomach, or jaw pain. Current data suggest that smoking, diabetes, and high triglyceride levels may increase the risk of heart attack more for women than for men. Women also are more likely to suffer from depression and sleep problems, both of which have recently been linked to heart disease. Research is ongoing to identify other ways women are different from men and explain why these differences exist.

One of the most noticeable gender differences is that **women tend to develop the first obvious symptoms of heart disease about 10 years later than men do,** usually around the time of menopause, typically the mid-40s to mid-50s. Because women tend to have lower levels of harmful LDL cholesterol, higher levels of HDL cholesterol, and more elastic arteries, it was thought that until they go through the hormonal changes of menopause estrogen provides a natural protective effect against heart disease. This conclusion led to the hope that hormone replacement therapy could reduce the risk of heart disease for women.

Results from the Women's Health Initiative and the Estrogen-Plus-Progestin Study that ended in 2002, however, showed that hormonal replacement therapy did *not* prevent heart disease and in fact could *increase* the risk of coronary events and stroke. It isn't clear whether estrogen actually protects against damage or only acts to mask the signs that disease is developing over the years, but scientists are continuing to investigate the link. (See page 121 for more information on the use of hormone replacement therapy.)

Thanks to general improvements in risk awareness, diagnosis, and treatment, the overall death rates from cardiovascular disease have declined about 25 percent since the 1990s. However, death rates in women haven't improved as much as they have in men. Several factors may explain this discrepancy. Some women may not be aware of the warning signs or report their symptoms early enough to be treated, or when they do, they may not be treated as aggressively as men are, especially if they are older women. In some cases—perhaps more than we realize—the higher death rate may be due to the fact that doctors have not been able to detect that these women had heart disease in the first place.

In some cases, common diagnostic tests may not be as accurate in

The American Heart Association and Your Doctor

Fighting heart disease in women is the job of a lifetime—for you *and* for your healthcare provider.

There was a time, not too long ago, when the public and the medical community weren't fully aware of women's risk for heart disease. Awareness has improved, but we still have a long way to go.

Advances in medical research in the past few years now mean we doctors have better ways to treat women with heart disease—and we also know that heart disease is highly preventable.

Cardiovascular disease is the leading cause of mortality among women, accounting for 37 percent of all deaths among females. Its public health impact is not related solely to mortality because advances in science and medicine allow many women to survive heart disease. For example, more than a third of women in the United States, or 41.3 million, are living with some form of cardiovascular disease.

In fact, all women are at risk for cardiovascular disease, underscoring the importance of a heart-healthy lifestyle for everyone, according to the American Heart Association's guidelines for prevention of heart disease in women. Based on the most current science and expert consensus, these guidelines were first issued in 2004 and then revised in 2007 to help healthcare providers make the best decisions about how to care for you and your heart.

The latest American Heart Association recommendations to physicians and healthcare professionals include these important updates for prevention of heart disease.

- Lifestyle changes are highlighted to help manage risk factors, including weight control, increased physical activity, alcohol moderation, sodium restriction, and an emphasis on eating whole grains, fruits, vegetables, and fat-free and low-fat dairy products.

- To help women quit smoking, counseling and nicotine replacement or other forms of smoking cessation therapy are recommended.

- Women should do the equivalent of 150 minutes or more of moderate-intensity activity (e.g., brisk walking) each week. One way to achieve this goal is to get at least 30 minutes of activity on most days of the week.

- Hormone therapy and selective estrogen receptor modulators (SERMs) are not recommended to prevent heart disease in women.

- Antioxidant supplements (such as vitamin E, vitamin C, and beta-carotene) should not be used for prevention of heart disease.

- The use of aspirin to prevent stroke depends on a woman's age and the balance between benefits and risks and should be determined in consultation with a physician.

LORI MOSCA, M.D., PH.D.

Professor of Medicine, Columbia University Medical Center,
Director of Preventive Cardiology at New York-Presbyterian Hospital,
and lead author of the Expert Panel/Writing Group for the American Heart Association
Evidence-Based Guidelines for Cardiovascular Disease Prevention in Women

women as previously thought. Angiography, for example, is considered very effective in locating obstructions in the larger main arteries. For the blockages typically found in men, angiograms work well to identify heart disease. In some cases, however, women with all the signs of a blockage undergo angiography that shows their arteries are "clear." These women are then considered to be at low risk for heart attack, but they continue to have symptoms that lead to repeated hospitalizations and tests, and ultimately may have a heart attack.

The difference in the accuracy of these angiograms can be explained by findings of the Women's Ischemia Syndrome Evaluation (WISE), begun in 1996. In this study, researchers found that plaque can accumulate and spread out smoothly and evenly on the linings of women's smaller arteries. These tiny arteries lose their ability to relax and dilate as needed. This condition, called coronary microvascular disease, reduces oxygen flow to the heart and results in symptoms similar to those of blocked main arteries. Because standard angiography focuses on the larger arteries, it cannot detect these problem areas. Coronary microvascular disease may affect up to 3 million women in the United States—and may explain why death rates from heart disease have not improved as much in women as in men in the past 30 years.

Most of the information known about coronary microvascular disease comes from the WISE research. Further ongoing studies are being conducted on better ways to detect and treat coronary microvascular disease, and on the role hormones play in the development of heart disease. As a result of these and other important studies specifically focused on women, both doctors and patients are realizing that they need a new set of rules when thinking about heart disease in women.

For example, a study evaluating the **effectiveness of lifestyle changes on heart health found that women responded better than men, even when the women did less to change their diet or to add exercise.** Another recent study indicates that arterial plaque may break down more easily in women's arteries than men's in response to appropriate lifestyle changes, perhaps because of differences in the way women's bodies use calcium. These findings suggest that women have even more to gain by making lifestyle changes to manage risk and protect their heart health throughout their lives.

As research continues, the medical community is beginning to respond to women's health needs. Doctors are redesigning their resources to suit women better—from the size of stents used to open up blocked arteries to the hardware used for valve replacement—and changing the way they ask questions in the examining room. Doctors are reevaluating their approaches to testing, diagnosing, and treating women with all forms of heart disease. (For more on diagnosis and treatment, see Chapter 10.) Certainly, as a woman, you will benefit from the recent increase in the attention paid to women's health, and in the years to come you will have access to better medical care developed specifically for women.

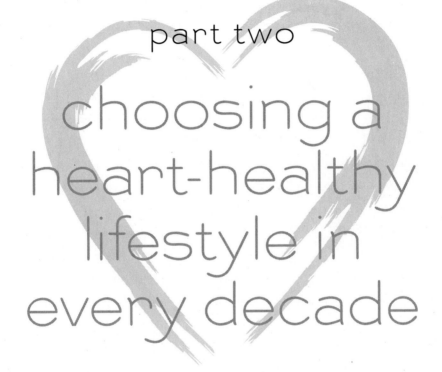

part two

choosing a
heart-healthy
lifestyle in
every decade

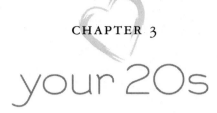

CHAPTER 3

your 20s

. . .

Me? Heart disease? It never occurred to me . . . then my grandmother died last year from a heart attack. When I found out the rest of my grandparents also had died from heart disease, I remember thinking, "Wow, I must be at risk." I've always worked out but only because I wanted to look good, not because I thought I was doing something good for my heart. —KRISTI, 27

. . .

t's never too early for you to adopt a heart-healthy lifestyle.

If you are between 20 and 30 years old, the **preventive steps you take now will have far-reaching consequences on your heart health throughout your life.** Although your risk of dying from heart disease in your 20s is very low, you may be already developing the risk factors that can lead to disease later in life. A wealth of new information and scientific research has alerted women to their risk for heart disease and heart attack: now is your chance to take advantage of both your youth and this new science to minimize your own risk.

Your lifestyle is made up of everyday choices—what you eat and how physically active you are, whether you smoke, drink alcohol, or use birth control pills—all of which can have a major impact on your long-term health.

Start making heart-smart choices today and every day:

- **Establish healthy eating patterns** and identify some healthy food and beverage options for your grab-and-go lifestyle and the party scene.

- **Remember that your body is keeping score.** You may be able to work off excess calories from junk food and calorie-laden beverages to control how you look on the outside, but a steady diet of unhealthy fats and sodium will gradually damage your arteries.

- **Learn about your family's health history** to determine whether you're at increased risk for heart disease. This is especially important for African American and Hispanic women, who are genetically predisposed to some risk factors for heart disease.

If you and other young women act on the heightened awareness that heart disease is largely preventable, your generation could be the healthiest one yet.

introduction

Your 20s are a challenge. You're trying to get your life started. You're making big choices, some with long-lasting consequences, and you're trying to have a good time. You're probably not thinking about the health of your heart.

But you should be. **Many of the choices you make now will have a long-term impact on your health,** so be sure your heart is on your list of priorities, along with finding a way to earn a living, picking a life partner, and deciding where to live.

You face lifestyle choices every day—what to eat and whether to work out, smoke, drink alcohol, or take birth control pills—and many of them may impact your heart. These daily choices can be life changing, and they deserve the same attention as other long-term decisions, such as investing in real estate or establishing a retirement savings plan. Everyday choices that are good for your heart are a long-term investment in your overall health.

Socializing often plays a large role in the 20s lifestyle, which can make sustaining healthy habits more of a challenge. Snacking and daily high-calorie coffee drinks, eating out, smoking, and drinking alcohol are typically part of the social scene. You are young, and you feel your body will bounce back from almost anything you do. That's somewhat true, since your youth does give you more stamina and resilience. If you continue to make unhealthy lifestyle choices over time, however, you may be setting yourself up for serious health consequences later on. **Your body keeps score, and the effects of your choices add up, even if the results don't become apparent for decades.**

It's Never Too Early

Your health may not be a big concern for you right now, but **your 20s is a good time to start thinking about what's going on with your heart and cardiovascular system. Heart disease is not just a man's disease or an old person's disease**—it does not discriminate based on gender or age. In fact, diseases of the heart kill more women in the United States than all cancers combined. Even in your 20s, you are still vulnerable to acquiring the risk factors that can lead to heart disease later. Some of those risk factors begin developing as early as childhood. For example, the artery-clogging plaque that can lead to a heart attack has been found in women still in their 20s. That's why caring for your heart and reducing your risk factors—even in your 20s—is so important. The equation is simple: the more you put your heart at risk, the greater your likelihood of heart disease and even heart attack. Just remember that the reverse also is true: **heart disease is largely preventable.**

Important research has identified that **lifestyle choices such as poor diet, lack of physical activity, smoking, and drinking excessive amounts of alcohol are controllable risk factors for heart disease.** You have the tools to get a jumpstart on preventing heart disease by eating properly, working physical activity into your life, not smoking, and drinking only moderately if at all. It is up to you to take action to reduce your risk: make heart-smart choices early in life to increase your odds of living a life free of heart disease.

Although you still have youth on your side, it's important to know that most risk factors for heart disease develop gradually and without outwardly noticeable signs. Ongoing physical changes that threaten your heart, such as rising blood pressure or high cholesterol levels, can begin early, but they also can be slowed or stopped with smart lifestyle changes. Armed with a thorough understanding of what to choose and why, you can make positive lifestyle decisions to establish lifelong patterns and habits that will help maintain a healthy body for the decades ahead.

Making Your Health a Top Priority

If you are like many other 20-somethings, you live for the now, postponing decisions about things that may offer big benefits later on, such as retirement plans and preventive health care. The downside is that "later" has a way of coming around much sooner than you expect, and previous unwise or unhealthy decisions do catch up with you.

Instead of waiting, make it your priority to embrace a healthy lifestyle now. Take steps to drastically reduce your risk factors for heart disease by eating a well-balanced diet, participating in regular exercise, avoiding cigarette smoke, and limiting your alcohol intake—plus visiting your healthcare provider for annual checkups. *Now* **is the time to stop any unhealthy tendencies so they don't become lifelong patterns.** The sooner you get busy focusing time and energy on making a healthier you, the better.

Your heart-health priorities for your 20s are to:

- **Pay attention to what you eat.** Establish a healthy eating pattern that you can sustain.

- **Adopt a regular exercise routine.** Make it part of your daily life so it becomes a lifetime habit. Find an activity you enjoy and have fun doing. You'll keep your heart healthy and avoid many of the risk factors for heart disease, as well as improving your fitness level, energy, and mental outlook.

- **Manage your weight.** Aim to develop a positive body image and take pride in caring for your health. Watch for the triggers, such as stress or depression, that make you vulnerable to weight gain.

- **Check your family history for risk factors**. If you are at risk for heart disease, educate yourself and talk with a healthcare professional about what preventive steps are right for you.

- **Schedule regular annual checkups.** Even in your 20s, it's important to get baseline measurements for blood pressure, cholesterol, heart rate, blood glucose, and weight so you can track changes in the future.

- **Don't smoke.** Avoid exposure to secondhand smoke as well.

- **Be aware of how social situations affect your lifestyle choices.** These include eating, drinking alcohol, and dangerous behaviors such as doing drugs. Choose the healthier options most of the time to protect your long-term health.

- **Choose your birth control method carefully.** Keep your heart health in mind, talk to your doctor about your options, and carefully weigh the risks against the benefits. Consider the health advantages—and disadvantages—of different birth control methods.

establishing healthy eating patterns

When your life is in high gear and you are trying to do it all, eating a balanced, healthy diet may not be a top priority. Research shows that women in their 20s try new fad diets, grab fast-food meals on the go, and rely on convenience foods more than they did in their teens. If this sounds like you, chances are you find it difficult to maintain a nutritionally sound eating plan. If you are concerned about your weight, you may be so focused on the calories you consume that you don't pay attention to providing your body with adequate nutrition. Calorie balance is important for healthy eating, but it is only part of the equation. Likewise, **if you rely on fast food and convenience foods, you may be eating too many unhealthy fats and too much sodium, as well as depriving your body of the important nutrients it needs** for you to function at the top of your game.

Healthy Food, Healthy Body

Science has demonstrated a direct connection between what we eat and how healthy we are. If you live on fast food or convenience products and feel healthy, you may not totally buy into that link. If you are not overweight or obese, you may ask what all the fuss is about. However, you may actually not be as healthy as you feel and look. Many restaurant and packaged foods contain high levels of saturated and trans fats, cholesterol, and sodium—all of which have a negative effect on your cardiovascular health. That's why it's important to have an eating plan that is both calorie-conscious and nutritionally sound. **Being aware of the quality of the food you eat as well as the quantity will help you find the right balance for overall good health.**

You will greatly improve your odds of being—and staying—well if you eat well. In turn, eating well means achieving a good balance from a variety of food groups by choosing nutrient-rich foods most of the time and limiting nutrient-poor ones. When deciding what foods and eating plan to choose, rely on known and trustworthy sources for information that has sound scientific research behind it and read the nutrition facts and ingredient lists on labels. Don't get caught up in marketing hype targeted especially to young adult women and in advertisements for the newest "superfoods" or the sure-fire diet or pill that guarantees weight loss. New products appear every day on the Internet, pop-up ads, dedicated food and health TV stations, and TV infomercials. With so many sources of information, it can be especially confusing to figure out which foods are right for your body and how they could affect your heart health. Remember the adage: if it sounds too good to be true, it usually is.

Set yourself up for good eating habits by following a well-balanced eating plan that includes all the essential nutrients from the following basic categories:

- **A wide variety of vegetables and fruits.** The more types of vegetables and fruits, especially deeply colored ones, you eat, the more likely you'll be to get a full spectrum of the vitamins and minerals, plus the fiber, your body needs. Based on a 2,000-calorie diet, you should aim for about five servings of vegetables and four servings of fruit every day. Bump up your daily servings with a banana at breakfast, an apple or a handful of grapes for a snack, and a salad of dark leafy greens as part of your lunch. A number of fruits, such as bananas, apples, grapes, and peaches, and vegetables, such as carrots and tomatoes, come in their own "packaging," making them great grab-and-go foods for a busy lifestyle.

- **Fat-free and low-fat dairy products.** As a young woman, you need plenty of calcium for strong bones, and consuming fat-free and low-fat dairy products is an ideal way to get this important nutrient. Simply pouring some milk into your morning coffee won't cut it: look for ways to get at least two to three servings every day. Fat-free or low-fat yogurt, cheeses, and larger amounts of that milk you used in your coffee are versatile and easy to include as part of quick meals or as snacks. For breakfast, try fat-free yogurt sprinkled with walnuts and berries, and for lunch perhaps low-fat Swiss cheese on whole-grain bread. Fat-free cottage cheese with diced peach or tomato would make a good snack with a double nutrition boost.

- **Whole-grain and high-fiber foods.** Refined grain products such as hamburger buns and white bread are made with flour that has had the nutrient-rich germ, or kernel, removed. For better nutrition, instead try whole-grain breads and pastas, as well as brown rice. Branch out with other grains you may not be as familiar with, such as barley and quinoa. Aim for about 25 grams of fiber a day, with at least half that amount coming from whole grains.

If you are pregnant, avoid eating fish with the potential for the highest level of mercury contamination, such as shark, swordfish, king mackerel, or tilefish. If family and friends fish in local lakes, rivers, and coastal areas and want to share their catch with you, check local advisories about the safety of the fish. Eating a variety of fish will help minimize any potentially adverse effects due to environmental pollutants.

- **Fish, especially those rich in omega-3 fatty acids.** Each week, include at least two 3-ounce (cooked weight) servings of fish. Fish that are high in omega-3 fatty acids, which have been shown to reduce the risk for heart disease, are especially good for you. These fish include tuna, trout, and salmon.

- **Lean poultry and meats.** In your 20s, you need about 60 grams of protein a day. You could eat 3 ounces of cooked skinless chicken breast (24 grams) at lunch and 3 ounces of cooked lean steak (26 grams) at dinner, filling in with 8 ounces of fat-free yogurt (9 grams) at breakfast or as a snack. Choose skinless white-meat poultry and lean cuts of meat to keep harmful saturated fat to a minimum.

- **Legumes, nuts, and seeds.** For fiber and meatless protein, include legumes, such as beans (not green beans, which are vegetables), peas, peanuts (and peanut butter), and lentils, in your diet. Most nuts, such as almonds and walnuts, are rich in heart-healthy unsaturated oils and when eaten in moderation and without added salt make good hunger-buster snacks that give you energy, not empty calories.

- **Healthy unsaturated oils and fats.** Replace fats that are high in saturated fat, trans fat, and cholesterol, such as butter and stick margarine, with unsaturated vegetable oils, such as olive and canola, to help keep down blood cholesterol levels. All fats are high in calories, however, so use them sparingly.

There is no wonder food or super food group. For overall good health, **you need a variety of foods that provide a broad range of nutrition.** If you leave out any of the food groups, you also leave out important vitamins, minerals, and other nutrients. In addition to concentrating on what to eat to maintain good health, also be aware of the less nutritious foods you might be eating too much of. These may include fast food and convenience and packaged foods, which often are high in saturated fat, trans fat, cholesterol, and sodium, the dietary villains that trigger reactions in your body that can lead to health problems later.

In addition to knowing what foods to include in your diet, it's important to know what to limit. To help you gauge how certain foods fit into your daily eating plan, use these general guidelines as you make your food choices.

- Aim to limit sodium to less than 2,300 mg each day. (If you are African American, you are more sensitive to sodium, so aim for less than 1,500 mg.)

- Aim to limit cholesterol to less than 300 mg each day.

- Aim to limit saturated and trans fats as much as possible. Try to be sure that your intake of these harmful fats does not reach an unhealthy proportion of your daily calorie intake.

IF YOU USUALLY EAT THIS MANY CALORIES EACH DAY					
	1,200	**1,500**	**1,800**	**2,000**	**2,500**
Keep **saturated fat** to less than	9 grams	11 grams	13 grams	15 grams	19 grams
Keep **trans fat** to less than	1 gram	1.5 gram	2 grams	2 grams	2.5 grams

Good Planning Leads to Better Nutrition

Before you begin to make any dietary changes, take a few minutes to assess your current eating habits—and be honest with yourself. Create an electronic food journal online or on your computer, or use the sample food diary page in Appendix C, to record everything you eat and drink for a seven-day period. Next to each item, make a note of the calories involved, the time of day, and whether boredom, peer pressure, or anything else besides hunger led you to eat. At the end of the week, look for patterns and evaluate your results. Do you eat too much junk food or fast food with little nutritional value? Are you an emotional or impulsive eater? Do you often eat at restaurants? Do you eat well during the day only to gorge on chips and dip at a party or at home late at night? Keep in mind that each seemingly small choice you make now will have an impact on your heart health later.

Once you've completed your review, you may find that you need to make only some minor tweaks to eat better. Perhaps you just need to remind yourself that ordering fast-food tacos one day will affect the overall balance of your diet during the week. Maybe, though, this exercise was an eye-opener, and you realize you need an extreme eating makeover.

Whatever your situation, decide how you can make changes both when you eat out and when you eat at home. Here are some strategies that can help you keep on track nutritionally when dining out:

- Identify and **order healthier menu options at your favorite restaurants.** If possible, review the menu online and decide in advance what you can order that will both satisfy your tastebuds and nourish your body. Then you will be less likely to opt for the not-so-healthy foods that may tempt you in the restaurant. For instance, at your favorite Asian restaurant, try the brown rice and steamed dumplings instead of the calorie- and fat-laden fried rice and egg rolls.

- **Avoid high-calorie beverages** that are low in nutritional value. Soft drinks, for example, provide you with about 200 calories in 12 ounces but no nutritional benefit. Instead order water with lemon or lime wedges for a flavor boost.

- To avoid too-large entrée portions, **make a meal of healthy appetizers.**

- **Consider ordering fish** as one of your staple dishes when you eat out, especially if you prefer not to cook it yourself.

- When you find yourself at the fast-food counter, **check out the salad options or grilled chicken sandwiches.** Be sure the salads you choose are not higher in calories and fat than the cheeseburger you're trying to replace! Salad dressing and toppings such as whole-milk cheese, bacon, regular mayonnaise, and "secret" sauces will add the calories, saturated fat, and sodium you want to avoid.

- If you grab fast food because you're in a hurry, **try your grocery store instead for healthy meals to go,** including soups, sushi, and salads. Prepared dishes are quick to pick up, and most stores offer several healthy options.

Dining at home allows you to control exactly what you are eating. When you're in the grocery store, however, you may be confused about what foods are actually wholesome. Conflicting messages and health claims advertised on many food products can make it hard to know what to choose. Keep in mind that foods that are processed for easy preparation and long shelf life usually contain more fats, sodium, and sugars. Read the nutrition facts panel on foods when you shop and compare brands to make the best choices. The majority of the packaged foods are found in the inner aisles of the grocery store; choose the bulk of your foods from the perimeter of the grocery store, where fresh fruits and vegetables, meats, fish, and dairy products are located. Here are some other strategies for good nutrition choices at home:

- For a quick dinner, **try prepared supermarket foods that aren't overly processed,** such as a prepared rotisserie chicken. Add instant brown rice and vegetables from your freezer and you have a quick, healthy, and balanced meal. For another meal, eat the leftover chicken in a salad with fruits or raw vegetables and a handful of nuts or between slices of whole-wheat bread.

- **Plan to cook fish at least once a week.** It's quick and easy and provides you with essential omega-3s, especially if you choose tuna, trout, or salmon. You can also buy salmon or tuna in cans or pouches and toss it into a green salad or whole-wheat pasta dish.

- **Plan ahead and cook in bulk one night a week.** Then you can enjoy ready-to-go meals at home instead of cruising the drive-through window.

- **To include a wider variety of vegetables and grains** in your eating plan, eat smaller amounts of your entrée and "accessorize" your meals with three or four side dishes. Take advantage of pre-cut, prewashed vegetables for quick and easy options, and buy small containers of prepared healthy salads and vegetable dishes.

- **Keep the freezer stocked** with a variety of fruits and vegetables without added sauces.

- Make it a point to **try a new vegetable or fruit frequently.** Visit farmers' markets for local produce. Explore new flavors; you may find you love foods you've never tasted before.

- **Boost your calcium intake** with nondairy foods such as fortified ready-to-eat cereals and tofu.

- If you crave a favorite fast food, such as pizza or a cheeseburger, **challenge yourself to replicate it at home with healthier ingredients.** Your version will almost certainly be lower in fat, calories, and sodium.

- **Keep snacks such as nuts, trail mix, raw vegetables, and fruit with you** when you're on the move. Having something healthy to munch close at hand will decrease your need to stop for a less healthy snack while you are out.

- **Include a small handful of nuts or seeds** in your salad, in your oatmeal or cold cereal, or in a snack-size plastic bag for an on-the-go snack. Because nuts are high in calories, limit yourself to no more than 1½ ounces (about twenty-three almonds, for example) on four or five days of the week.

- When you crave high-calorie sweets, reach instead for a handful of berries. Deeply colored berries are full of fiber, vitamins, and natural antioxidants, and since they're not full of processed sugar, they'll satisfy your craving without making your blood sugar surge and then crash. **Buy fresh berries** and divide them into snack-size plastic bags or containers that can go in your purse, briefcase, or backpack.

Eating well *can* be part of a 20s lifestyle. Don't wait until later to create healthy eating habits: good habits are as easy to keep as bad ones. Remember that your overall goal is to **eat a good balance of healthy foods *most* of the time.** You don't need to be perfect and you don't need to give up the foods you just can't live without. If you want a juicy cheeseburger with all the trimmings, go ahead and eat it—every now and then. Once you establish your healthy eating pattern, you'll be on your way to a healthier future.

establishing an active lifestyle

Are you an active 20-something woman, with an exercise routine that's a regular part of your daily life and your interactions with friends? If so, you are one of the many women working out at the gym, running or biking, taking yoga or dance classes, rock climbing, playing on a softball team, or training to run in a marathon or fundraising race.

On the other hand, regular physical activity may not be part of your lifestyle. Perhaps you were active as a teen but your habits have changed. The time you spent on exercise when you were in college or living with your parents may now be taken up with other responsibilities, such as working a full-time job, raising children, and/or taking care of a home. **Yet your 20s are exactly when it's important to make physical activity a regular part of your life.** If inactivity has crept into your lifestyle, it has become a new risk factor for you for heart disease. The good news is that **inactivity is a *controllable* risk factor.** By including physical activity in your regular routine, you take that control and reduce your risk. You don't have to run marathons or even join a gym. Just 30 minutes a day of a moderate activity such as brisk walking can get you started.

Why Exercise Is So Important to Your Heart

If you are physically active, do you exercise to look good, feel good, or control your weight? All of these are common and valid reasons, but did you realize that **regular physical activity also provides valuable benefits to your heart?** Research shows that regular aerobic exercise will reduce your chance of developing high blood pressure, high cholesterol, diabetes, and obesity—all major, yet controllable, risk factors for heart disease. When you are active enough to raise your heart rate, you decrease the amount of adrenaline in your body. Less adrenaline means more-relaxed blood vessels, a slower pulse, lower blood pressure, and, ultimately, less strain on your cardiovascular system overall. In addition, exercise reduces the amount of harmful LDL cholesterol your body produces and helps boost the helpful HDL cholesterol, which in turn will help keep your arteries clear of plaque. You can see that being physically active really does affect your health in a big way.

In addition to directly benefiting your heart, moderately intense or vigorous exercise gives you more energy, makes you feel better about yourself, reduces the effects of stress, encourages more-restful sleep, and delays the effects of aging. **An ongoing exercise routine also will:**

- help you develop greater endurance and strength

- tone, strengthen, and lengthen muscle

- increase flexibility

- improve circulation and increase the delivery of oxygen and nutrients to your body's cells

- help you lose or control weight

- boost confidence and elevate mood

Exercise Your Options

Here are some ideas on how to make physical activity part of your lifestyle:

- **Make a list of the physical activities you enjoy most,** then circle one or two that you are going to find time to work into your lifestyle. Chances are you won't stick with an activity if you don't like doing it.

- **Let the energy of others motivate you.** Turn a physical activity into a social one so you can be with friends and get fit at the same time. Popular workout choices include hip-hop or salsa dancing, spinning classes, "boot-camp" programs, kick-boxing, and even belly dancing.

- **Try joining a local gym to fight boredom.** The gym allows you to exercise in a social setting and offers a variety of options that can range from basic aerobics to yoga and Pilates, from racquet-ball to indoor rock climbing and swimming.

- If you prefer to work out away from the public eye, try some of the hundreds of workout DVDs offering a multitude of approaches. **Use fitness technology to your advantage** with electronic dance simulators and gaming stations. All these options can provide you with a totally in-house workout.

- **Get adventurous** and get involved in snowboarding, skiing, skating, surfing, hiking, or mountain biking. They're all great forms of physical activity that let you enjoy the great outdoors.

For an option that is inexpensive and can be done almost anywhere, with or without a partner, **try brisk walking!** It doesn't require equipment other than a good pair of walking shoes, can be done in a safe environment (including the mall or in your office complex), and is a proven aerobic workout. To make the most of your walk time, follow these pointers:

- Wear a pedometer for a week to measure how many steps you take in an average day. If you're in the *not active* (2,000 to 4,000 steps per day) or even *moderately active* (5,000 to 7,000 steps per day) category, look for ways to gradually add more steps to your daily routine. Maybe you'll like walking so much you'll end up with at least 10,000 steps per day, categorized as very active.

- As you walk, keep your stomach muscles pulled in and your back straight. Swing your arms and maintain good form.

- Walk on softer surfaces, such as asphalt, smooth dirt and grass, and treadmills, to reduce the impact on your hips, knees, and ankles. Sidewalks tend to be the hardest on your joints.

- Try to walk at least 30 minutes at least five days a week. If that's too much for you now, start with just 10 or 15 minutes daily. Next week, increase the time by 5 minutes daily, and so on until you reach the goal of at least 30 minutes per day.

- Improve your endurance by walking a little faster each week. A brisk pace (or moderate intensity) is about how you'd walk if you were late for an important meeting.

- Take several short walks instead of one long one if they are easier for you to fit into your day. Short sessions of 10 minutes each can add up to the same health benefits as one long session.

- Get a boost from your mp3 player. Studies show that you'll walk longer and harder if you listen to music as you walk.

- Combine walking with weight training to burn calories and strengthen your bones.

If you often travel for business or pleasure, walking is a good exercise option as long as you pack walking shoes and follow a safe route. Many hotels offer workout rooms, or you can bring along your own portable equipment and exercise in the comfort of your room. Workout DVDs, resistance bands, jump ropes, and a doorway bar take up little space in your suitcase but give you a lot of flexibility to fit in your fitness regimen whenever it's most convenient for you.

Go for the Goal

What constitutes a reasonable workout for you? Look for activities that include a cardiovascular workout, which means something that involves moving large muscles, such as those in your legs, with enough intensity to noticeably increase your heart rate. Moderate-intensity aerobic activity should make you feel like you do when taking a brisk walk (you can talk but not sing); vigorous-intensity should make you breathe rapidly and substantially increase your heart rate, as when running (you can say only a few words without catching your breath). **The recommended goal for cardiovascular fitness is at least 150 minutes** (2 hours and 30 minutes) **of moderate-intensity or 75 minutes** (1 hour and 15 minutes) **of vigorous-intensity aerobic physical activity each week.** You can also combine moderate and vigorous activities to suit your schedule and preferences in order to reach an equivalent total. Aerobic activity should be performed in episodes of at least 10 minutes, and preferably it should be spread out through the week. For example, you could:

- walk at a brisk pace for 30 minutes a day two days a week, then jog for 20 minutes on two other days.

- walk briskly for 30 minutes on five days a week.

- spend 30 minutes in a step aerobics class of moderate difficulty five times a week.

- walk briskly for 30 minutes on two days, spend 60 minutes dancing at moderate intensity one evening, and spend 30 minutes once a week mowing the lawn (moderate intensity).

- work out to a vigorous aerobic exercise program, either in a gym or following a DVD or downloadable video, for 20 minutes four days a week.

- spend 30 minutes a day dancing on an electronic dance pad set on moderate difficulty five times a week.

In addition to aerobic activity, you should include strength training (also called resistance training) for each muscle group about twice a week. By putting strain on the bone, weight-bearing exercises help maintain or even increase bone density. Activities such as lifting weights, hiking, jogging, or playing racquet sports can increase bone mass and delay the onset of osteoporosis.

When you're young, you may feel up for anything, so it might be tempting to abuse your body in your enthusiasm for results. You could, however, be left with chronic injuries. Like fad diets, arduous and over-the-top exercise crazes that you can't sustain won't do much for you in the long run. Establish a reasonable ongoing routine that matches your capabilities; it will serve you better and longer.

Whether you work out with friends or on your own, **setting a personal goal or taking on a challenge is a big motivator.** For example, sign up for a run that's just beyond your comfort zone and then use the training period to stretch your limits. If you aren't ready to go it alone, check out an online Couch-to-5K running program. Designed to transform you from couch potato to runner, these programs get great results because they detail exactly what you need to do, one step at a time, to train for a specific goal.

Also become aware of how you are standing or sitting. Remember to "pull up and in" and resist the tendency to slump over. Techniques such as those used in Pilates, ballet, and yoga focus on a strong center and are helpful in regaining good posture and a tighter belly, especially after pregnancy.

As well as toning your body, exercise has physiological effects that improve your emotional well-being. When you use large muscle groups, you get your blood pumping and increase the oxygen flow to cells throughout your body. In response to prolonged, continuous exercise, your body produces endorphins, hormones that induce a feeling of well-being and reduce the negative effects of stress. These rewards add greatly to the quality of your overall health and lessen your need for unhealthy coping mechanisms such as overeating, excessive alcohol use, or smoking.

Take advantage of your youth to participate in the many interesting, dynamic, and fun sports and other activities available to you. Take joy in what your body can do, and gear up your mind-set to maintain a workable exercise routine throughout your 20s. **Set the stage *now* for an active and healthy lifestyle** that lasts through your 30s, 40s, 50s—and well beyond. You'll not only look good but also keep a healthy heart.

> Get comfortable with your body and appreciate the fact that unless you have atypical health issues, it's young and strong. Recognize what you like best about yourself, decide to be healthy, and capitalize on your assets. It's important to reach a healthy weight for your height and body type, but being fit and healthy is not the same as being thin. (For more information on the ideal body weight range for you, see Appendix C.) It's quite possible to be skinny and unfit at the same time!

managing your weight

If you are like most other young women, when you look in the mirror you probably are thinking more about how your body looks on the outside than how it looks on the inside. If looking good is your motivation for managing your weight, that's okay. The important bonus is that you are keeping extra weight from threatening your heart health. But not carrying extra weight does not mean your habits are necessarily heart-healthy. For instance, you may eat what you want, when you want, and how much you want—and then exercise like crazy the next day or so to work it off—and that might work for a while, but it isn't sustainable. In addition, **your body will keep tabs on your lifestyle choices in ways you can't see,** such as eventual increased blood pressure or plaque in your arteries, before you notice any extra weight gain.

Alternatively, you may still eat the way you did when you were a teenager, but without being as active as you were then. Lots of women in their 20s transition from an active lifestyle that might have included walking on campus, playing sports with friends, or frequent dancing to a relatively sedentary lifestyle that can include sitting for hours in an office and collapsing in front of the TV at night. If this shift has happened to you, those unburned calories will start to add up to unwelcome weight gain unless you make some adjustments.

Stop the Bulge Before It Becomes a Battle

The eating patterns you establish in your 20s are likely to be the ones you carry into your next decades, so it's important to develop healthy habits now. Your metabolism is running fairly high in your 20s, but it will begin to gradually slow down in your 30s and your body composition will change from mostly muscle to more fat. To avoid future weight gain, **you'll need to take in fewer calories and be more active as you age.**

Even with the typically high-powered metabolism of your 20s working for you, you can't count on your youth to protect you against weight gain. No matter what your age is, if you eat more calories than you burn, you will gain weight—and it doesn't take much to tip the balance: **an extra 100 calories every day will add up to 10 pounds of weight gain in a year.** As you get older, it will become more and more difficult to lose that extra 10 pounds, so now is the ideal time to get in the habit of making every calorie count toward maintaining a healthy weight.

Balancing Calories In with Calories Out

How can you manage your weight in a healthful way? The answer is simple: **balance the calories you take in with the calories you burn.** If you already have extra weight that you want to lose, you'll need to find a better balance between the calories you consume and those your body uses. The healthiest way to lose weight is to cut back on high-calorie foods while being sure that you are getting adequate nutrients. That way the foods you eat will give you the greatest nutritional payoff. To lose weight, first determine how many fewer calories you need to consume and how many more you need to burn each day. (To find out how many calories a day you should eat to maintain your current weight, see the box on page 253.) Remember that weight loss is best sustained through a gradual process. You didn't gain the weight overnight, and you can't expect to lose it overnight.

Next, make a plan that focuses on your losing 1 to 2 pounds a week; stay away from any fad diet that promises unrealistic results or isn't nutritionally sound. To identify how your eating and exercise habits are contributing to your weight, keep a record of everything you eat and your physical activity for one week. Write down every meal, snack, and drink, including the amount and approximate calories for each. (Check for calorie values on product packages, in recipes, and by searching online, such as on the USDA nutrient database.) Also, write down all the ways you are physically active during the week, such as "30 minutes jogging" or "10 minutes walking the dog." (Use the food and activity diary templates in Appendix C.) Once you have one week's information recorded, review it and analyze your current eating and exercise patterns. If your eating habits provide good nutrition and balanced calories, you're on a healthy course. If, however, you notice unhealthy patterns, such as too much junk food, mindless munching, late-night high-calorie splurges, or too much time on the couch, you should reassess and plan for healthier alternatives. When you're deciding between the deep-dish pizza and the grilled chicken salad, for example, think about how you're going to "spend" your daily calories and what the payoff will be. Look for choices that will give you the most for your "nutrition budget"; go for the foods that are high in nutrients and low in calories. Foods that are high in empty calories, such as sodas and many desserts, aren't a good health investment.

The best predictor of whether you can avoid gaining excess pounds or keep off what you've lost is how much you regularly exercise. In the previous section, you read about the benefits of physical activity and about the amount you need for heart health. If you are actively trying to lose weight, you need to step up your daily amount of exercise. To lose weight effectively and keep it off, you may need 60 to 90 minutes of daily moderate-intensity activity. If that seems like too much, start with what's realistic for you. Start with a short walk—at least 10 minutes—every day and gradually work up to your goal. Try a quick office workout, which can include pushups against the edge of your desk (either sitting or standing), leg raises, and lifting weights while you sit in your chair. **Some exercise is always better than no exercise,** with every bit of activity adding up to help you subtract pounds!

It's a common belief that *all* you have to do to lose weight is exercise harder without paying attention to what you eat, but consider the facts. The reality is that 20 minutes of moderate exercise burns only about 100 calories. That's an hour and a half of brisk walking for every typical cheeseburger! If you're eating too much of the wrong high-calorie foods, it would be impossible to exercise enough to burn off the extra calories. Remember, it's all about balancing how many calories you eat with how many your body uses.

Try these common-sense approaches to managing your weight in a healthy way:

- Train your brain to think, **"Quality first, then quantity."** Choose a wide variety of foods that give you the best chance of eating all the nutrients you need.

- **Learn what a reasonable portion of different foods should look like.** (For example, one serving of pasta should be about the size of a baseball.) If your typical portion is larger, cut back.

- **To lose weight, eat only 75 percent of the amount of food you normally eat, or substitute lower-calorie foods for the high-calorie foods you eat regularly.** For example, if you are used to buying a cinnamon roll on your way to work, try toasting a cinnamon-raisin English muffin at home instead and save yourself about 300 calories.

- Test your calorie sense and **become aware of the calories in the foods you eat,** especially those you consume on a regular basis.

For instance, you might be surprised to find out the calorie count in many popular blended coffee drinks. A whole-milk, cappuccino-type beverage with whipped topping can be as high as 500 calories.

- Combine strategies: eat smaller portions on one day, substitute lower-calorie for higher-calorie foods on another, and follow a reliable prescribed eating plan when you need a jump-start to lose a few pounds. **Switching tactics will help keep you from getting bored with your weight-loss plan.**

- **Drink a glass of water before meals** to help fill up, or have a broth-based soup to start your meal.

- **When you eat out, plan ahead to take half your meal home.**

- **Stay away from all-you-can-eat buffets** and pass on the bread or chips offered before many restaurant meals.

- **Watch out for mindless munching.** Before you snack, stop and think whether you're really hungry, rather than thirsty, bored, or feeling blue.

- **Anticipate cravings and stock up on healthier alternatives.** Keep fruit, fat-free yogurt, microwave popcorn, or snack-size bags of nuts in the office to satisfy your snack attacks.

- **Know your triggers** for needing comfort food. Replace the food with a distraction and something else that gives you satisfaction, such as a walk, a hot bath, or a new coat of nail polish.

- **Plan ahead for late nights** out on the town. Stock your freezer with lower-calorie healthy entrées so it will be easier to stay away from the fast-food drive-through window when you come home hungry.

- **Make time for your favorite physical activities or find new ones that fit into your schedule.** Spend time being active with friends. Think up fun adventures such as taking a daylong hike or bicycle trip to a favorite or new destination.

Take advantage of the energy and vitality of your 20s to stop creeping weight gain and to get and stay lean and healthy. With some simple planning and the commitment to stay in control of your weight, **you can avoid the yo-yo dieting that so many women turn to as they get older.** Make it your habit to eat well and stay active—you'll feel better, look great, and establish a heart-healthy lifestyle that will keep you in shape through your 20s and the decades ahead.

managing your health care

If you're in your 20s now, **you're part of a truly fortunate generation of women.** It is only in your lifetime that scientists have come to learn more about heart disease specifically in women. That research has resulted in potentially lifesaving information for women your age, and you have decades ahead of you to use it to make a real difference in your heart health care. Unlike your mother and grandmothers, you have the advantage of knowing your risk for heart disease and heart attacks, so you can be proactive in your own care. **Heart disease does not automatically come with aging, and it is largely preventable.** It's up to you to make the decisions to eat well, exercise regularly, maintain a healthy weight, establish ongoing relationships with trusted healthcare professionals, and do everything else you can to reduce your risk factors for heart disease.

Find Trusted Healthcare Providers

To set the stage for good long-term health care, **it's important *before* you have a medical issue to find healthcare providers you trust.** Although you may feel well today, you still need regular screening tests so you and your doctor can establish baseline records and monitor your health. (See Appendix A for a health screening checklist.) Have you established a comfortable and ongoing relationship with a primary-care physician? If not, make that your first step. Be sure to schedule regular well-woman visits, and discuss how your individual risk factors affect the big picture of your overall health. Your healthcare provider should check the basics, which include your weight, height, heart rate and rhythm, and blood pressure. She or he should check and record your weight and blood pressure at every visit so patterns or changes that develop over time can be tracked. For instance, even in your 20s, you are not immune from developing health issues such as high blood pressure. If you are monitoring your blood pressure now, any increases that remain constant can be treated early enough to prevent serious damage.

Your healthcare provider should also listen to your heartbeat and to your lungs as you breathe, check for signs of developing disease such as unexpected swelling in your legs and ankles or changes in the blood vessels at the back of your eyes. Your 20s is also an ideal time for a blood test to determine your lipid profile, which measures the levels of LDL and HDL cholesterol, triglycerides, and other blood fats.

Be proactive about your health. Keep a written or computerized record of all your test results for your own reference. As you get older or when you change healthcare providers, you'll want to refer to your health records to monitor for developing risk factors. If you do develop a health condition that needs managing, you will also need those records to make better-informed decisions about medication or treatment.

Managing Risk Factors in Your 20s

Remember that *all* women are at risk for heart disease. In addition to the risks posed by being physically inactive and obese or overweight, other areas of concern to manage in your 20s may include birth control, smoking, and drinking. Be sure to mention to your healthcare providers anything that might influence your medical situation and your risk for heart disease, including your family history. (For more information on these risk factors and others, see Chapter 2.)

FAMILY HISTORY

Now is the best time to **investigate your family's health history.** The sooner you ask your older relatives about their health issues, the more likely you are to get information before memories fade or family members die. As with the color of your eyes, tendencies for certain health conditions can be passed from one generation to another. If you have a blood relative who had heart disease at an early age (for example, a heart attack or stroke before age 55 for men or age 65 for women), your risk increases significantly. Risk factors such as high blood pressure, high LDL cholesterol, low HDL cholesterol, and diabetes also tend to develop within families. As you learn about your family's health history, record it and keep the document in a safe place with your other personal medical records. (For a template of a family history tree, see Appendix D.) Be sure to share this information with your healthcare provider and discuss what it means for you. (For more information on genetic predisposition, see page 15.) The more you know about your family's health history, the more you can do to reduce your risk of heart disease.

ORAL CONTRACEPTIVES

Research has found that birth control pills are linked with increased blood clotting in some women, particularly if they smoke. Although today's low-dose oral contraceptives carry a much lower risk of heart disease and stroke than earlier ones did, women who take birth control pills and also smoke or have high blood pressure are at higher risk for developing blood clots and having a heart attack. That's why **women who smoke should not take birth control pills.** Every woman should ask her healthcare provider to measure her blood pressure before prescribing oral contraceptives, then have her blood pressure checked regularly.

SMOKING

Smoking can be a large part of the 20s social scene. Smoking may seem fun and "cool" now, but it is the number one most preventable risk factor for heart disease and, as you now know, heart disease is the number one killer of women. In fact, studies have shown that **smoking is still the single most important factor accounting for heart attacks in younger people.** The message is simple: **if you smoke, stop** *now,* especially if you are taking oral contraceptives. Smoking is also an addictive habit, and the sooner it is broken, the better. Cigarettes aren't the only form of tobacco that's dangerous to your health; so is secondhand smoke. (For further information on smoking, see page 21.)

EXCESSIVE ALCOHOL USE

The adverse health effects of regular excessive drinking and binge drinking are more dangerous for women than for men. Excessive drinking (an average of more than one drink per day for women) can raise blood pressure and lead to stroke; contribute to obesity, high triglycerides, cancer, and other diseases; and cause heart failure. Although you might see reports of research suggesting that drinking *moderate* amounts of alcohol may protect your heart, the American Heart Association does not recommend that nondrinkers start drinking alcohol to seek health benefits. **For women, a *moderate* amount of alcohol means no more than one drink per day on average.** One drink means a 12-ounce beer, 4 ounces of wine, 1.5 ounces of 80-proof spirits, and 1 ounce of 100-proof spirits. Drinking too much can have destructive effects that may not take their toll in your 20s or even your 30s but may well catch up with you in your 40s and 50s if the behavior continues. The physical consequences won't be as easy to shake off as you get older. If you do drink alcohol, be aware of what you drink, how much, and how often, and be aware that the drinking habits you develop today may stay with you for the decades ahead. (For further information on alcohol and its effects on women, see page 24.)

• • •

While you're young and feeling full of life, it may seem unnecessary to focus on keeping up that vitality. The truth is, though, that you actually can do something now that will pay you back for years to come. Your young age does not keep you immune from having or developing risk factors for heart disease. Although the medical community can offer you many resources for good health care, *you* have to take the initiative to take advantage of them. Don't wait until you're older to think about your heart and the quality of life you want to have in middle age and beyond. Take responsibility for your own heart health by making good decisions today for a healthier future.

checklist for achieving heart health in your 20s

✓ **Talk to your family members** to learn about their health history and record it.

✓ **Make it a priority to get healthier,** especially if you plan to have children.

✓ **Learn to count nutrients,** not just calories.

✓ **Establish a plan to make** healthy eating and regular exercise part of your regular routine.

✓ **Follow the plan** and modify it if necessary.

✓ **Keep your weight at a healthy level,** particularly if you are considering becoming pregnant.

✓ **Balance your calories in with your calories out.**

✓ **Find trusted healthcare professionals.**

✓ **Get regular health checkups.**

✓ **Be aware of and manage your risk factors**—especially taking birth control pills, smoking, and drinking—and discuss these with your healthcare professionals.

Pregnancy and Heart Health

When you are pregnant your circulatory system undergoes functional changes to allow blood to circulate through the placenta and nourish the baby. One important change is in *cardiac output*, which is the amount of blood that the heart pumps each minute. During pregnancy, cardiac output increases by about 30 to 40 percent. Your heart rate and total blood volume also increase, and your blood pressure may decline slightly because more of your blood is being directed to feed the uterus, kidneys, and skin. These adjustments are normal and designed to supply the developing baby with blood that provides oxygen and nutrients.

The demands on your circulation continue to increase during pregnancy, diminishing slightly at about 10 weeks before delivery and increasing again just before labor and delivery. Your circulation returns to normal about two weeks after the baby is born. Symptoms such as swollen ankles, increased tiredness, dizziness, and frequent urination are all normal temporary results of these changes in your heart and circulation.

Even with a normal heart, during pregnancy you may experience these cardiovascular abnormalities, as well as other complications.

- **High blood pressure:** Gestational high blood pressure (hypertension) is a serious complication of pregnancy. About 8 percent of all pregnant women develop hypertension, most often after the twentieth week. That's why you should have your blood pressure checked often throughout your pregnancy. Also, if you have problems with your blood pressure while pregnant, your risk of developing high blood pressure after pregnancy is significantly increased. Be sure to have regular checkups.

  Very high blood pressure can occur, along with rapid weight gain, swollen ankles, and protein in the urine. This disorder is known as *preeclampsia*, or toxemia of pregnancy. It affects the blood vessels, kidneys, liver, and brain. Preeclampsia can also cause decreased blood flow through the placenta, leading to

continued

slower growth, or even loss, of the fetus. Although preeclampsia can be treated, it requires immediate medical attention and often necessitates a preterm delivery. If left untreated, it can progress to a life-threatening condition called *eclampsia.* Visual disturbances, severe headaches, and abdominal pain usually precede eclampsia.

Heart murmurs: In the course of your prenatal checkups, your healthcare provider may detect a heart murmur when listening to your chest. The extra blood flowing through your heart causes this new sound. Usually this doesn't indicate that anything is wrong with your heart. Rarely, however, a new murmur can mean that there's a problem with a valve.

Arrhythmias: *Arrhythmia* means the heart beats out of rhythm or too fast or slow. Arrhythmias can develop for the first time during pregnancy in a woman with a normal heart or as a result of previously unknown heart disease. Occasionally, arrhythmias are noticed when a healthcare provider measures the pulse. Most often, there are no symptoms and no treatment is required. Sometimes arrhythmias can cause palpitations, dizziness, or lightheadedness, and, rarely, fainting.

Some women develop a form of diabetes during pregnancy called *gestational diabetes.* If you are diagnosed with this condition, you are at higher risk for developing diabetes. Be sure to follow up with your healthcare provider yearly to check your fasting blood sugar level so he or she can detect changes over time that could indicate you are developing type 2 diabetes.

If you are overweight or obese and thinking of having children, try to lose the weight *before* you become pregnant to avoid the risk of added complications for you and your baby. Talk with your healthcare provider or perhaps a nutritionist about how to develop an eating plan that will be best for both you and your baby, both before and during your pregnancy. More important than focusing on losing weight is establishing a balanced eating pattern that will form the basis of the healthy eating habits you pass on to your children.

your 30s

. . .

I try to exercise every day and make healthy food or walk the extra block to pick up a healthy meal. Little changes make a big difference. There are so many things you can't control, but exercising and eating right are things you *can* control. It can be daunting to think, "Wow, exercise 30 minutes a day? I don't even get 5 minutes for myself." But you realize that being active not only gives you more energy but also a whole new outlook on life. —LORAINE, 35

. . .

You're busy—really busy—but don't be too busy to take care of yourself.

Most women in their 30s struggle to balance working with having the personal life they want—one that includes enough time for family, friends, and themselves as well.

With so much going on, who has time to worry about a heart-healthy lifestyle? You do! Your health should be a top priority. **If you can reach 50 without developing the major risk factors for heart disease, you could live your *entire* life without heart disease.** That's a goal worth striving for!

To make your heart health a priority:

- **Start managing your weight now,** if needed. It's not going to get any easier.

- **Make sure exercise is on your to-do list or daily planner.** Think of it as "your time," whether you enjoy it in solitude or share it with a friend.

- **Monitor your numbers.** It's important to have baseline measurements for your blood pressure, blood cholesterol, and heart rate as part of your medical profile.

Establish heart-healthy habits now that will last a lifetime!

introduction

Your 30s are a definite "rush." You may be focused on finding and nurturing a relationship with a lifetime partner, building and advancing a career, and perhaps starting and raising a family. Juggling these priorities makes it difficult to find the work-life balance that's right for you.

Many women in their 30s find that taking care of themselves is the first thing that "comes off the list." It's hard to find time for a bubble bath, let alone for the planning needed for a heart-healthy lifestyle of nutritious eating and physical activity.

But don't neglect yourself. **Paying special attention to your heart health is a priority you should commit to in this decade.** Why now, when you are probably the busiest you've ever been? Because heart disease risk is real and starts early, and you can take steps to reduce that risk. You may think you needn't worry about being a statistic until you are older, but heart disease—even heart attack and stroke—does happen to women in their 30s. Now, **when you are young and healthy—*before* risk factors have accumulated to dangerous levels—you have the** most power to greatly reduce your odds of having heart disease or stroke in your later years. Heart disease is *not* an inevitable part of aging; you can identify your risk and make changes to your lifestyle to fight back. What you do now to protect your heart can add years of better health and increased vitality to your life.

Understanding How Your Body Is Changing

If you feel well and have no symptoms of serious illness, it's easy not to focus on your health right now. However, heart disease doesn't wait until you are in your 30s or even in your 20s—your risk can start to increase even in childhood. In fact, healthcare providers recently have found accumulations of harmful plaque in the arteries of girls in their teens or younger! Your body has been absorbing, recording, and reacting to everything you've experienced until now. In other words, your body has kept tabs on what you have put in it and what you've done to it. **By your 30s, there's a good chance that you have already developed some potential threats to your heart.**

Certain changes that occur in your circulatory system during pregnancy also can cause stress on your heart. (For more information, see the special section on pregnancy and heart health that precedes this chapter.) In addition, you may find the extra after-baby weight particularly difficult to shed, and those unwanted pounds can pose a risk to your overall heart health.

When you are in your mid-30s, another physical change affecting your weight is the slowing down of your body's metabolism. If you're like most other women about your age, you'll start losing a quarter of a pound of muscle or more every year and gaining at least that much in fat. With this metabolic change comes the increased chance of weight gain. If you don't keep that weight gain under control, it can lead to overweight or obesity—a major risk factor for heart disease.

Making Your Health a Top Priority

What if you could reach middle age without developing the major risk factors for heart disease—high blood pressure, high cholesterol, obesity, and diabetes? Science suggests that **if you can do this**—and it is possible—you will have only an 8 percent risk of developing cardio-vascular disease. On the other hand, if you do develop two or more of these risk factors by middle age, you will face a 50 percent lifetime risk—that's a significant difference! These major—yet controllable—risk factors are heavily influenced by your lifestyle now. For example, your decisions on what to eat, whether to smoke, whether to drink alcohol, and how much to exercise have a cumulative effect on your body's meta-bolic processes.

If taking your health seriously hasn't been one of your priorities in the past, make it one now. In fact, by doing so **you might even be able to reverse the effects of poor choices you may have made in your 20s,** and you'll decrease your chances of having health problems later. You *can* make more time to care for yourself, but you have to commit to it. Don't let the day-to-day frenzy of your life distract you from taking stock of your lifestyle and its effect on your body and long-term quality of life. Just as you invest time and energy in your family, friends, and job, you should do the same for yourself and your health.

You need realistic strategies to make your lifestyle a healthy one. You don't have to be a superwoman. As you face each day, **focus on the important things you can control, such as eating well and exercis-ing. You can start small:** each day eat at least one balanced meal and schedule two or preferably three 10-minute walks. The idea is to find regular routines that fit well within your personal lifestyle. *Now* is the time to stop any unhealthy tendencies—eating meals haphazardly, over-eating, being sedentary, and procrastinating about seeing your health-care professional—from becoming lifelong patterns. The sooner you get busy focusing some of your time and energy on a healthier you, the better!

Your heart-health priorities for your 30s are to:

- **Commit to taking care of your health *now*.** The decisions you make today will have a significant effect on your heart health in the decades to come.

- **Develop a nutritious eating plan.** Choose foods that nourish your body and meet your personal caloric needs. Eating healthy is something that you can control and that has a great impact on your heart health.

- **Add physical activity to your schedule.** If you keep on top of your weight and muscle tone now, it will be easier to stay fit in your later decades.

- **Establish a healthy weight and maintain it.** It's easier to keep excess weight off now than to lose it as you get older and your metabolism slows.

- **Record your family's health history.** Find out about your family members' health history from your parents and grandparents. Review the information and analyze it for patterns. Note any existing risk factors for heart disease. If you are at risk, talk with a healthcare professional about what preventive steps are right for you.

establishing healthy eating patterns

Now that you're in your 30s, it's a good time to assess your eating habits. If your overall eating pattern could use a makeover, recognize that and challenge yourself to start fresh. **Make the 30s the decade that you commit to better eating.**

To help keep your heart disease risk low, **develop and maintain a personal eating plan that provides your body with good nutrition,** which in turn will both minimize your risk and supply you with the energy you need to better cope with life's demands. Rather than letting the hectic pace of your 30-something life dictate what and when you are going to eat, take back some control by finding ways to include nourishing meals in your everyday routine. A haphazard eating approach can lead you off course and directly into a nutritional ditch! As is true for most things in life, you'll need a good plan of action to get on the right path. By following a healthy eating plan, you will be en route to a healthy heart!

Healthy Food, Healthy Heart

Your 30s may be one of the most demanding and trying decades of your life. No matter whether you are climbing the corporate ladder in your career, enjoying life on your own, raising a family, traveling for work or pleasure, or any combination of these, you are most likely a busy woman on the go. Feeding your body properly is especially important when you're busy and under stress. You may be eating plenty of food, but unless you're getting the right balance of nutrients from a variety of food groups, your body isn't getting what it needs to be healthy, energetic, and in peak condition. **Your eating plan goals should be focused on nutrient-dense foods,** such as vegetables, fruits, and whole grains, and to steer away from foods that are high in saturated and trans fats, cholesterol, sodium, and added sugars.

The basic aspects of a healthy diet include:

- **A variety of colorful vegetables and fruits.** The more variety you fit into your diet, the wider the range of nutrients—including vitamins, minerals, and fiber—with which you will reward your body. Choose the vegetables and fruits that are deepest in color: the deeper the color, the higher the level of nutrients. Based on a 2,000-calorie diet, you should aim for about five servings of vegetables and four servings of fruit every day. (And don't pretend that finishing the green beans on your toddler's plate gives you a full serving of green vegetables!)

- **Whole-grain and high-fiber foods.** These foods provide essential vitamins, minerals, and, especially, fiber, which plays an important role in heart health by helping lower harmful LDL cholesterol levels. Good sources of whole grains can be found in whole-wheat breads, whole-wheat pasta, brown rice, and whole-grain cereals. Also give bulgur and quinoa a try. At least half your grain servings should be *whole* grain. If you buy a prepared grain product, check that the labels list a *whole* grain as the first ingredient. High-fiber foods include beans, fruits, and vegetables. To include more high-fiber foods, you could start the day with oatmeal and blueberries and have an unpeeled pear as a midafternoon snack, for example. On average, aim for about 25 grams of fiber a day.

- **Fish rich in omega-3 fatty acids.** Studies have shown that omega-3 fatty acids in the diet reduce the risk of coronary artery disease. Make it a goal to eat fatty fish, such as salmon, tuna, and trout, at least twice a week. Consider making a point of ordering fish when you eat out. Another option is to buy tuna and salmon in a can or pouch and enjoy it in a salad or in a whole-wheat pita for lunch. If you're concerned about the mercury in fish and shellfish, remember that the health risks from mercury exposure depend on the amount of seafood eaten and the levels of mercury in the individual fish. Eat a variety of fish to minimize possible adverse effects. If you are pregnant, planning to become pregnant, or nursing—or if you're feeding the fish to young children—avoid the fish most likely to have mercury contamination, such as shark and swordfish. In most circumstances, however, the benefits of eating fish far outweigh the risks.

- **Fat-free and low-fat dairy products.** Dairy products provide calcium for good bone health and are essential during pregnancy. You should consume two to three servings of fat-free or low-fat dairy products to get the usually recommended amount of between 1,000 and 1,200 mg of calcium each day. Ask your healthcare professional how much calcium is right for you, however. For example, you can reach 1,000 mg by drinking 1 cup of fat-free milk (300 mg) and eating 8 ounces of fat-free yogurt (450 mg) and 1 ounce of soft goat cheese (250 mg). Fortified ready-to-eat cereals, greens such as spinach and kale, and some legumes and soybean products also provide calcium.

- **Lean poultry and meats.** Your body needs protein but not as much as you might think. In fact, Americans tend to eat too much protein, and that can actually leach calcium from your body. Aim for no more than about 6 ounces of cooked lean, low-saturated-fat poultry or meat (8 ounces before cooking) each day. For a well-balanced dinner that keeps your protein needs in perspective and emphasizes some of the other foods you need, visualize a plate divided into fourths, with two sections for vegetables and fruits, one for grains or starchy veggies, and one for a protein.

american heart association
complete guide to women's heart health

- **Legumes, nuts, and seeds.** Legumes, such as peas, beans, lentils, and peanuts (including peanut butter), are a great source of fiber and meatless protein. It's a good idea to try to eat at least one vegetarian meal each week, and legumes can be the base for many nutritious options. Nuts and seeds also provide fiber, protein, and healthy unsaturated oils, but use them sparingly because of their high calorie content.

- **Healthy unsaturated oils and fats.** Vegetable oils such as olive and canola provide heart-healthy unsaturated fats. When part of a diet that is also low in saturated fat and cholesterol, unsaturated fats may help keep down blood cholesterol levels.

As you develop your eating plan, be sure to include several healthy choices from all these food groups to ensure that you get maximum nutritional value and don't feel deprived.

In addition to knowing what foods to include in your diet, it's important to know what to limit. To help you gauge how certain foods fit into your daily eating plan, use these general guidelines as you make your food choices.

- **Aim to limit sodium to less than 2,300 mg each day.** (If you are African American, you are more sensitive to sodium, so aim for less than 1,500 mg.)

- **Aim to limit cholesterol to less than 300 mg each day.**

- **Aim to limit saturated and trans fats as much as possible.** Try to be sure that your intake of these harmful fats does not reach an unhealthy proportion of your daily calorie intake.

IF YOU USUALLY EAT THIS MANY CALORIES EACH DAY					
	1,200	1,500	1,800	2,000	2,500
Keep **saturated fat** to less than	9 grams	11 grams	13 grams	15 grams	19 grams
Keep **trans fat** to less than	1 gram	1.5 gram	2 grams	2 grams	2.5 grams

Good Planning Leads to Better Eating

Before you begin to create a new eating plan, conduct a quick, informal self-assessment of what you eat now—and be honest with yourself. Are you eating healthy foods on a regular basis? Do you eat too much junk food or fast food with little nutritional value? Do you need to lose some weight? Are you eating foods that provide you with the best health pay-off? Are you eating too many foods high in saturated and trans fats, cholesterol, and sodium?

Next, record your current eating habits for a week, writing down *everything* you eat and drink. (There's a sample food diary at the end of Appendix C.) Next to each item, make a note of the meal or time of day and whether you ate because of anything besides hunger, such as stress or depression. At the end of a week's time, look for patterns and evaluate your results. Are you eating the recommended amounts of vegetables, fruits, and grains each day? What do you need to cut back on, and what should you eat more of? Are you an emotional eater?

Once you complete your evaluation, you most likely will make some eye-opening discoveries. Maybe you will be pleasantly surprised to find that you need to make only small modifications to eat better. On the other hand, maybe you will conclude that you need an extreme eating makeover. We have some tips that will help you, regardless of whether your eating plan needs fine-tuning or an overhaul.

Now that you know what you should be eating, you need to fit healthy eating into your busy schedule. Is healthy eating really more time-consuming than unhealthy eating? No, but you do need to be a better planner so that you'll be more successful in following through on your good intentions. Let's say you haven't planned for dinner. You could easily end up ordering takeout food, going to a drive-through window at a fast-food chain, or preparing packaged frozen foods with too much sodium and too much saturated fat. Buying lunch in your company's cafeteria, out of the office vending machines, or at a restaurant you pass while doing errands can be easy and convenient choices during a hectic day, but choosing one of these options is probably less heart-healthy than planning ahead and bringing lunch from home after stocking your fridge with quick and easy healthy options.

Eating well does take planning, organization, and time management skills, especially at first, but the earlier you get started, the more easily you can establish new healthy habits. It's a good investment to decide on menus, make a grocery list, and shop once a week. With the ingredients waiting in the refrigerator and a plan in place, you'll be able to have dinner on the table in the same time it takes to visit the drive-through. You'll get added value if you're feeding a family, because serving healthy meals sets a good example for your children to follow.

The challenge for you is to find the best ways to minimize time spent on grocery shopping and cooking so you can enjoy nutritious meals on at least most days. Keep these makeover strategies in mind as you develop your eating plan:

- **Establish a repertoire of several healthy meals you enjoy that are easy to make.** Standardize your grocery list so you'll always have the ingredients for these meals on hand. Even when you are pressed for time, you'll have what it takes to make a healthy meal.

- **Keep on hand at least three good-for-you and palate-pleasing snacks,** such as low-fat string cheese, unsalted nuts, and frozen grapes. When you need a munchie, you'll be prepared with something healthy.

- **Start a monthly meal exchange program with friends and neighbors.** Once a month, prepare a healthy recipe that makes enough for two dinners. Freeze one at home and meet with the group to swap the other. You'll come home with a different freezer-ready entrée to add to your supply.

- **Buy meats or other protein sources that can be used for several meals during a week.** Bake more chicken breasts than you need for dinner, saving the rest to use in enchiladas, homemade soups, and chicken salad. Cook enough black beans for a meal plus enough to add to salads, tacos, and vegetable soup.

- Short on time? **Keep individually wrapped fish fillets in the freezer.** They defrost in minutes, so they're fast and easy to cook.

- **Slip vegetables** such as spinach and grated zucchini **into soups, stews, and meatloaf** when you don't have time to prepare a separate side dish.

- **Bump up your calcium intake** by drinking smoothies and eating creamy sauces and soups made with fat-free yogurt. Nondairy sources of calcium include fortified ready-to-eat cereals and tofu.

- **Find ways to incorporate supernutritious grains,** such as quinoa, into your meals. Substitute brown rice and whole-grain pasta for their white counterparts, and remember that corn counts as a whole grain.

- **Make a grocery list of the staples you need to restock,** and add all the ingredients you'll need for the recipes and snacks you've chosen for the week.

- To maximize time, **shop for food only once a week** and make your trips as efficient as possible.

- **Focus your shopping on the perimeter of the grocery store,** where you'll find the produce, meats, and dairy products. Avoid the processed foods usually found in the center aisles.

- Once you're back home, pack your favorite raw veggies, such as baby carrots, in resealable snack-size bags. Keep them in the fridge to grab and go. **Prep vegetables in advance so they're ready for use** in weekday dinners.

- **Buy fruit that travels easily,** such as apples, bananas, and grapes. These make great portable snacks for work or to share at your kids' soccer games.

- **If you drink whole milk, ease into fat-free** by buying 2%, then 1%, and, finally, fat-free so your taste buds will adapt. For an even more gradual switch, combine some whole milk with some 2%, then continue to change the proportions until your family is drinking only 2% milk. Continue this process until everyone is drinking 100% fat-free milk.

- **Keep fat-free cheeses in the refrigerator.** Snacks such as string cheese calm edgy appetites better than sugary snack foods and provide you with needed calcium.

- **Pack resealable snack bags of favorite heart-healthy cereals or healthy homemade trail mixes,** such as an ounce of unsalted almonds and whole-wheat cereal, as to-go snacks and a way to add fiber to your diet.

- **Network with other women** to see what works for them. Find a blog—or start one—to trade ideas with other women who are in situations similar to yours.

Don't let "I'm too busy" be the reason you don't eat as well as you should. Make it a priority and a commitment to provide the best and most healthful food for yourself and your family. Remember that it's not the occasional cheeseburger, but the overall pattern of your food choices over time that counts. If you can settle into a comfortable routine of choosing the healthy options most often, you'll be doing yourself and everyone who depends on you for their meals a nutritious favor.

establishing an active lifestyle

If "too busy" has become your slogan in your 30s, have you also used it as your crutch for not exercising? If so, do yourself a favor and move working out to a higher spot on your priority list, no matter how busy you are. **Consider the time you spend exercising as a gift to yourself rather than as a chore to be endured.** It's time that allows you to unwind, shake off stress, reenergize, and invest in a healthier middle age and beyond.

Exercise not only burns calories to keep your weight under control but also provides additional heart-health benefits, reduces stress, and improves self-esteem—all of which have long-lasting payoffs. If you already have an exercise routine—and kudos to you if you do—you may not even realize all the ways you're helping your body.

Why Exercise Is So Important to Your Heart

Personal trainers and physicians agree that **exercise is the number one form of preventive medicine.** Aerobic exercise reduces many of the risk factors for heart disease by improving levels of blood pressure, LDL cholesterol, triglycerides, and insulin sensitivity. In fact, studies have shown that a routine of regular moderate exercise in your 30s will help offset the metabolic processes that increase body fat and decrease muscle mass as you age. Staying one step ahead of a slowing metabolism will help you keep a healthier weight, bump up your energy level, and reduce your risk for disease.

An ongoing routine of moderately intense or vigorous exercise will:

- counteract changes in metabolism

- help you lose or control weight

- help keep blood pressure at a healthy level

- reduce harmful LDL cholesterol and increase helpful HDL cholesterol

- reduce the risk of diabetes

- help you develop greater endurance and strength

- tone, strengthen, and lengthen muscle

- increase flexibility

- improve circulation and increase the delivery of oxygen and nutrients to your body's cells

- boost confidence and elevate mood

Get Up and Get Going

With your busy lifestyle, you may be saying to yourself that adding time for a regular exercise routine is easier said than done, or you may believe you're already getting enough exercise—but **don't confuse *busy* with** *active*! Chasing a toddler or sprinting to the bus, however exhausting, is not a suitable replacement for a sustained exercise routine. Now that you are in your 30s, it's important to **structure your life to make exercise a priority** if you haven't already done so. Schedule time for it just as you would for any other important event, appointment, or commitment.

Before getting started, talk with your healthcare professional about the best ways to include both aerobic exercise and strength training in your personal lifestyle. Then make an honest assessment of how you spend your day, looking for pockets of free time—even 10 minutes—to set aside for yourself. Keeping a journal for a few days may help you find windows of opportunity when you can squeeze in some physical activity.

Next, set a long-term goal for yourself and break it down into smaller targets that you can accomplish in one workout session. For example, your goal might be to take a 5-mile walk by the end of this month. Today's target could be to walk the dog from your house to the park, which is one mile. This weekend's target might be to walk to the quick mart, about a mile and a half away, to pick up a newspaper. Once you've reached your goal, give yourself a new challenge. Consider running or walking in a local Heart Walk, or even training for a marathon! Use the activity diary in Appendix C to record your accomplishments.

Exercise Your Options

Here are some how-to tips and ideas for adding physical activity to your lifestyle:

- **Choose activities you enjoy and mix them up** so that you don't get bored. Walk with a friend or spouse, take a kick-boxing or tae kwon do class, dance to a DVD, or join an organized sports team. If you're a mom and need child care, consider joining a local health club or community activity center that offers babysitting services. Maybe you'd prefer to get up 30 minutes earlier several times a week to exercise before going to work or waking up the children. Jog in place or walk on a treadmill while watching a TV show you usually don't make the time to see.

- **Keep track of your efforts.** Note on your calendar or PDA every day that you exercise so you can easily see your achievements add up!

- **Use your PDA** to schedule reminders to get moving.

- **Choose a target goal and concrete benchmarks.** Reward yourself for your successes and don't dwell on what you couldn't get done. For example, decide that you will jog twice around your block every morning for one month. If you achieve your goal, give yourself a reward like a new pair of running shoes or a pedicure to mark the occasion. If you have to miss some days, just chalk it up as a temporary derailment and keep going.

- **Exercise even when you feel tired or simply don't want to—** the exercise will reenergize you.

- If you are a mom, incorporate ways to **get in physical activity with your children.** Consider playing tag in the park, swimming relay races, or pulling your kids in a wagon or pushing them in a stroller. If your young children's school is close enough, walk with them instead of driving. All of you will get some exercise, and it's a golden opportunity to talk.

- If you are single or new to an area, **think about social networking opportunities** that will allow you to meet people and incorporate exercise into your life. Look online for local running, walking, and bicycle clubs as well as community or workplace softball or soccer teams.

Go for the Goal

Whatever aerobic activity you choose to do, **your goal should be at least 150 minutes** (2 hours and 30 minutes) **of moderate-intensity or 75 minutes** (1 hour and 15 minutes) **of vigorous-intensity aerobic physical activity each week.** You can also combine activities to reach an equivalent total of moderate and vigorous activity. "Moderate intensity" means that as you are exercising, you notice that your heart rate increases. This level of intensity is comparable to walking at a speed of about 4 miles per hour. You should feel as if you can talk but not sing as you exercise. "Vigorous" means that the activity level should make you breathe rapidly and substantially increase your heart rate, and you should not be able to say more than a few words without catching your breath.

Aerobic activity should be performed in episodes of at least 10 minutes, and preferably it should be spread out through the week. For example, you could take a 30-minute brisk walk on five days each week. For variety, you could ride a bike on level ground (moderate intensity) for 30 minutes on two days, work out at a gym for 20 minutes at vigorous intensity on two days, and spend 30 minutes mowing the lawn (moderate intensity) on the weekend.

To get an accurate idea of your baseline activity level, try wearing a pedometer for a week, then determine how many steps you take in an average day.

- Not active = 2,000 to 4,000 steps per day

- Moderately active = 5,000 to 7,000 steps per day

- Very active = At least 10,000 steps per day

If you're in the *not active* or even *moderately active* category, look for ways to gradually add more activity to your daily routine. Many of the suggestions for filling in those available pockets of time work here, too. Even the simplest activities can add up to a more active lifestyle if you're moving energetically, and the benefits are cumulative, so it all counts toward your goal. That means that you can, for example, take three 10-minute walks during the same day if doing so fits your schedule better than one 30-minute session. Keep in mind that **it is the regularity, not the intensity, of activity that offers the most protective benefit for your heart.** If once in a while you get off track from your regular exercise routine, that's okay. Just be sure that the inactivity becomes more the exception than the rule.

In addition to aerobic activity, you should include strength training (also called resistance training) for each muscle group at least twice a week. By putting strain on the bone, weight-bearing exercises help maintain or even increase bone density. Activities such as hiking, jogging, or racquet sports can increase bone mass and delay the onset of osteoporosis. Also become aware of how you stand or sit. Remember to "pull up and in" and resist the tendency to slump over. Try classes in Pilates, ballet, and yoga to develop a strong center. All these techniques are helpful in regaining good posture and a tighter belly, especially after pregnancy.

As well as toning your body, exercise causes distinct physiological effects that improve your emotional well-being. When you use large muscle groups, you get your blood pumping and increase the oxygen flow to cells throughout your body. In response to prolonged, continuous exercise, your body produces endorphins, hormones that induce a feeling of well-being and reduce the negative effects of stress. In addition to counteracting stress, exercise gives you more energy, combats depression, and improves your sleep. These rewards add greatly to the quality of your overall health and lessen your need for unhealthy coping mechanisms, such as overeating, drinking too much alcohol, or smoking.

It's easier to stay motivated and stick with a long-term exercise routine if you take a positive approach and appreciate all the ways being active can help you, whether you're just getting started or have been active for years. Make it a priority to make exercise a part of your lifestyle, and enjoy better health for many years to come.

managing your weight

As a woman in your 30s, you probably have become adept at managing your responsibilities—at work, in your household, and elsewhere. You need to take that same responsibility for your own well-being and use the skill set—time management, good organization, and advance planning—that you use in other areas of your life to effectively manage your weight. *Now* is the time to put those practical skills to work for *you*—and your heart health.

Battling the Bulge in the 30s

The more hectic life is, the less likely you'll make nutritious food a priority and the more tempting it is to grab whatever food is available and worry about eating better "tomorrow." If the food you grabbed was high calorie and high fat, did you think, "I'll just have a salad for dinner," "I won't eat dinner tonight," or "I'll watch what I eat this weekend"? Stop feeling guilty and start channeling your energy toward developing a weight-management plan that gets you moving and grooving in your 30s.

Research tells us that the 30s is the decade when the pounds do start to pile on. **After age 30, American women often gain a pound a year.** That may not seem like a lot, but do the math. By the time you are 40, that's 10 extra pounds and by 50 that's a total of 20 extra pounds!

In your 30s, you may notice that you can't lose weight (especially those stubborn after-baby pounds) as quickly and easily as you once could. You're starting to experience the first signs of a slower metabolism, and your body doesn't need as many calories as it once did. A slower metabolism increases the body's shift from muscle mass to fat, making you more vulnerable to further weight gain. At the same time, fast food, lunch meetings, and perhaps even cleaning your kids' plates can undo your efforts to stay lean.

Another complication is that, thanks to the genetic legacy of our cave-dwelling ancestors, human bodies are programmed to keep stored fat as a defense against future famine. So by nature, we are working at odds with our own bodies. Even if you aren't eating a lot of food, you may have trouble losing weight and keeping it off if you don't exercise regularly.

In a culture obsessed with fashion-model thinness and manufactured beauty, it's almost inevitable that media images affect how you see yourself and what you might think of doing to look good. Although the way a flat tummy and small waist look on the outside may be important to you, the health risks of being overweight or obese in your 30s go much deeper. For example, an apple-shaped woman (with more weight at the waist than at the hips and thighs) is at greater risk for heart disease. That's why **keeping your waistline at 35 inches or less is so important.**

✓ The extra weight you carry now will increase your risk of heart disease.

✓ Being overweight increases your risk of developing diabetes.

✓ The more weight you gain now, the harder it will be to lose later.

The most effective and long-lasting way to manage your weight is to make sure that the calories you take in do not add up to more than you burn off. What does this mean? It simply means maintaining a healthy balance by eating well and exercising regularly.

Balancing Calories In with Calories Out

Keeping everything in your life balanced, especially your health and weight, takes effective management skills and follow-through. If you have fallen into unhealthy habits, whether recently or over the years, it's not too late to break them. With a little planning and determination, you can change to better eating patterns that work within your daily life. Before you know it, you won't have to think twice about what to eat— or what not to. Enjoying good food in reasonable portions can become second nature.

As your body changes, you'll need to **balance your daily food intake** (calories in) **with the energy your body is using** (calories out). To do this, you'll need to determine how many calories you should be consuming a day. (For information on how many calories a day you should consume, see Appendix C.) If you are at a healthy weight, keep up the good work by burning as many calories as you take in. If you need to reduce your weight, make a plan to decrease your calorie intake and increase your level of physical activity. In other words, eat less and exercise more.

Try these simple weight-control techniques.

- **Make breakfast part of your routine.** Breakfast revs up your energy level and keeps your metabolism going. Researchers have found that skipping breakfast is associated with a higher risk for obesity.

- Eat your usual diet, but **choose smaller portions of every food at every meal.**

- **Replace the high-calorie foods** you eat with lower-calorie substitutes. Try marinara sauce on pasta instead of the Alfredo.

- **Find family-friendly recipes** that everyone will love, so you can prepare one meal instead of two.

- **Develop an eating plan, and stick to it.** If you didn't include your kids' leftovers in the plan, don't finish what's on their plates. Those calories do count, even if you eat them standing in the kitchen!

- If your kids do eat dinner earlier than you, **enjoy a low-calorie salad while they are eating** so you can join them without being tempted to help them clean their plates.

- **Keep low-calorie healthy foods on hand,** such as baby carrots, fat-free yogurt, and cut-up fruit—frozen grapes are a treat!

- **Watch for liquid calories** in soft drinks, coffee concoctions, fruit juices, and alcohol. Try water or hot tea instead, and add a twist of lime or lemon for a flavor boost.

Research shows that the **women who are most successful at losing weight and keeping it off are those who make regular exercise part of their lifestyle.** The good news is that you don't have to lose every unwanted pound before your health will benefit. So start with a manageable goal. Studies have shown that **losing just 10 percent of your body weight may help reduce your risk for heart disease, stroke, and diabetes.**

You will lose weight by cutting calories, but the key to keeping the weight off is also to exercise. Exercise is essential to maintaining weight loss and muscle tone. You may even find that your appetite decreases after a workout. Strength training also helps prevent the muscle loss that may result when you drop a lot of pounds.

As we've said, managing your weight successfully takes a plan, just like managing other areas of your life; it doesn't just happen. To help yourself lose weight and keep it off, make time to eat well and to add a regular exercise routine to your lifestyle. **Keeping your weight under control is an important part of reaching middle age without developing many of the major risk factors for heart disease.** The long-term payoff will far exceed your efforts now.

managing your health care

In your 30s, you need a strong, resilient body to help you meet the physical demands of balancing the various aspects of your life. Therefore, healthcare issues in this decade are of prime importance.

Broaden Your Team of Healthcare Providers

If pregnancy and birth control have been major healthcare issues for you, you probably have established a good relationship with your ob-gyn. However, as you age, it's important to broaden your team of healthcare professionals to include a general practitioner as well. If you are unsure where to start, ask friends or family for recommendations, do research on reliable websites, or contact local hospitals or your insurance company for references. The person you choose for your primary medical care should make you feel comfortable discussing all aspects of your health. It's best to have a solid relationship in place *before* you have a health problem.

Once you have established your team of healthcare providers, be sure to speak with them about your medical history and the lifestyle choices you've made to date. (For advice on talking to your doctor, see Appendix B.) Be open and honest. Be sure to mention elective and cosmetic procedures such as dental surgery, breast implants, Botox, and skin peels. If you haven't already, discuss your family history and any existing factors you may have for cardiovascular disease. Remember that although certain factors such as heredity cannot be changed, the effect of these factors can be moderated by maintaining a healthy lifestyle. Your everyday lifestyle choices, such as whether to smoke or drink alcohol, also have a huge impact on your long-term risk.

As a woman in your 30s, **it's important that you begin to have regular annual checkups with your healthcare professional.** If you did not get baseline screenings for your blood pressure, cholesterol, and glucose in your 20s, get them now. (For more information, see Appendix A.) These screenings are important because they provide a way for you and your doctor to compare these numbers with new readings each year and identify any changes that might signal a potential problem.

Managing Risk Factors in Your 30s

All women are at risk for heart disease, and the more risk factors you have, the higher your risk. In addition to the risks posed by physical inactivity and obesity/overweight, the other areas you most likely will manage in your 30s include the health concerns that come with reproductive issues such as birth control and pregnancy. (For more information on pregnancy and heart health, see page 65.) If you smoke, you are adding a major risk factor.

SMOKING

Heart disease is the number one killer of women, and smoking is the number one preventable risk factor for it. Studies have shown that smoking is still the single most important factor accounting for heart attacks in younger people. It also seems to be riskier for women's hearts than for men's. A recent study found that women who smoke have heart attacks nearly 14 years earlier than women who don't smoke. The message is simple: If you smoke now, stop! Just as it is not too late to gain great benefits in your 30s from eating healthier and exercising routinely, it is not too late to reap rewards from stopping smoking. In fact, the risk of heart attack decreases quite quickly after quitting, dropping by half after just one year. If you need help to quit smoking, talk to your healthcare professional about cessation programs.

BIRTH CONTROL

Many women in their 30s are faced with birth control decisions. Some of these choices may have an impact on heart health. (For more information on oral contraceptives, see page 62.) If you are over 35, take oral contraceptives, and have other risk factors, especially if you smoke, your risk of developing blood clots and having a heart attack increases *greatly*. Talk to your healthcare professional about the safety and effectiveness of various birth control methods and discuss which may be the best options for you.

POLYCYSTIC OVARY SYNDROME

This common disorder of the endocrine system disrupts your normal hormonal cycle, sometimes causing pelvic pain or cysts. It's usually identified in women who have trouble conceiving in their 30s. Symptoms include obesity, increased waist measurement, insulin resistance, high blood pressure, higher levels of LDL cholesterol, and lower levels of HDL cholesterol—all of which increase the risk of heart disease. If you've been diagnosed with this condition, be proactive in your 30s by carefully monitoring your risk factors, eating a healthy diet, and being physically active on a regular basis.

· · ·

The 30s are busy years filled with vast opportunities and commitments. Women may be juggling home and career, raising a family, settling into a life with a partner, traveling the world, and perhaps even caring for aging parents. You are faced with many changes, big decisions, and hard work. To have energy for it all, **you must make yourself—and your health—a top priority.** Make the 30s the decade you give yourself the priceless gift of good health.

checklist for achieving heart health in your 30s

✓ **Take back some time** in your busy schedule for you.

✓ **Make it a priority to get healthier,** especially if you plan to have children.

✓ **Plan to make healthy eating and regular exercise** part of your routine.

✓ **Follow the plan** and modify it if necessary.

✓ **Keep your weight at a healthy level,** particularly if you are considering becoming pregnant.

✓ **Balance your calories in with calories out.**

✓ **Broaden your team of healthcare professionals** to include a general practitioner as well as an ob-gyn.

✓ **Get regular health checkups.**

✓ **Record your family members' health history.**

✓ **Be aware of and manage your risk factors**—especially birth control pills and smoking. Discuss these with your doctors.

CHAPTER 5

your 40s

. . .

I want women to know that their family history is important, that they should know their blood pressure and cholesterol numbers. Even though I have a family history of heart disease, I still didn't think that, as a woman, it could happen to me. If I had realized that I was at risk, I hope I would have lived differently. —THERESA, 41

. . .

For the first time since you were a teenager, your body is changing in major ways.

You're a "reverse teenager." Your dropping hormone levels are a reality. The onset of perimenopause, and ultimately menopause, will require some changes in your lifestyle choices.

Heart disease tends to develop about 10 years later in women than in men. Even so, each year in the United States, more than 9,000 women under 45 experience a heart attack. Though that's a relatively small number, it's just the tip of the iceberg for the eventual toll heart disease takes on women. That's why taking your own risk for heart disease very seriously is such an important step.

You can delay or even *prevent* the progression of heart disease by making lifestyle changes:

- **Eat for good nutrition—and eat a little less.** Reduce your portions as your metabolism slows.

- **Get or stay physically active.** If you can't jog as fast or as far as you used to, modify your expectations, but don't stop. Women lose 5 percent of their physical fitness each decade as they age. Getting active now can slow the decline markedly.

- **Be vigilant about checking for risk factors.** Schedule regular visits to your doctor, and if your blood pressure or cholesterol levels start to rise, take immediate action.

Your awareness that your risk of heart disease is real can motivate you to make positive lifestyle changes.

introduction

By the time you hit the big 4-0, you may well have noticed that you're just not as young as you used to be. Perhaps you are more aware of signs of aging in your body, such as having a little less stamina or a bit more trouble losing extra pounds.

Family milestones also may sharpen your awareness of growing older. Watching your children grow or your parents age and confront their own health issues may make you wonder what your own senior years might be like.

Whatever challenges and changes you experience in your 40s, just remember that you've got a lot of living to do! In fact, statistically, a 40-year-old woman in the United States has about half her life yet to lead. You still have plenty of time to make any lifestyle changes for better health and longevity and to improve the quality of the years ahead.

Understanding How Your Body Is Changing

Although you may be worrying about laugh lines and other outward signs of aging, taking care of your heart in your 40s is no laughing matter. You have reached the point in your life when your risk of heart disease becomes very real. If you could see inside your cardiovascular system, you might find signs of rising blood pressure or plaque lining your arteries—first steps in the development of coronary artery disease.

Just as your hair begins to show gray streaks in your 40s, your heart too is becoming vulnerable to the risk factors that come with age. That's why *this* **is the time to take care of your cardiovascular system and keep your heart muscle strong.** You can do a lot to lessen your chances of developing risk factors that pose an inherent threat to your heart health, but those risks go up if your lifestyle includes eating an unbalanced diet, being inactive, smoking, or other unhealthy choices.

Reaching 40 brings you closer to menopause and physical changes that can increase your risk of heart attack. Perimenopause, the long period of gradually reduced hormone production that precedes menopause, can start as early as your late 30s but generally occurs sometime in your 40s. Passing through the phases of perimenopause, with your levels of estrogen and progesterone rising and falling, can take from two to eight years. Lower levels of estrogen can affect your blood cholesterol levels, increasing harmful LDL cholesterol and decreasing protective HDL cholesterol. As estrogen gradually decreases, you also start to lose bone mass more quickly than you replace it, increasing your risk of osteoporosis. During this decade, you may develop elevated levels of blood pressure or your blood sugar levels may start to rise slightly. Emotionally, you may experience mood swings that affect your lifestyle choices without your even realizing it. (If you've ever *had* to have a chocolate bar without really knowing why, you might be able to blame it on hormones.)

Now that you are facing your 40s and these physical realities, it's important to understand that **heart disease is not something that affects only older women.** Just ask one of the many women who have survived a coronary attack or stroke in their 40s and she will tell you otherwise. You may feel and look great, but the statistics show that you cannot afford to take your current health for granted. Research shows that the conditions that significantly increase your risk of heart disease (discussed in Chapter 2 and at the end of this chapter) can begin as early as childhood, and they continue to develop and intensify with age.

By your mid-40s, you likely have some accumulation of arterial plaque that began long before you ever heard the word *atherosclerosis*. That does not, however, mean you are powerless to keep your risk level from increasing as you get older. In fact, quite the opposite is true.

Making Your Health a Top Priority

Statistics show that, being a woman, **if you reach your 50s without developing the major risk factors for heart disease, you face only an 8 percent risk of developing cardiovascular disease,** rather than the 50 percent lifetime risk you'll face if you have two or more risk factors such as high blood pressure, high cholesterol, obesity, or diabetes. With those odds, **it just makes good sense to work—or continue to work—at staying as risk free as possible.**

Another piece of great news is that according to current research, appropriate lifestyle changes may be able to stop or perhaps even *reverse* the buildup of arterial plaque in women. A recent study evaluating the effect of lifestyle changes on heart health found that women responded better than men, even when the women did less to change their diet or add exercise. Because you still may have half of your life—or more—ahead of you, it's time to assess your overall lifestyle patterns and make the changes needed to protect your heart to the best of your ability.

Your 40s present a golden opportunity to take charge and improve your health or recommit to the healthy lifestyle you may already be living. The first step is to educate yourself on the risk factors for heart disease in women. Heart disease is not inevitable, and you can take steps to reduce your risk or control risk factors. **The most actionable steps you can take with the biggest payoff are eating well, being physically active, and managing your weight.** By changing your unhealthy habits to healthy ones, you'll be better equipped to fight the major risk factors for heart disease, and you may be able to avoid or delay taking medications for conditions such as high blood pressure, high cholesterol, and diabetes.

Your family medical history also plays an important role in your risk for heart disease. Do you know enough about it to know how it affects your level of personal risk? If not, start by asking blood relatives to share their medical histories with you. If a parent has high blood pressure, for example, you should be especially careful to get regular checkups, watch your intake of dietary sodium, and exercise regularly. If your grandmother had a heart condition, do you know what it was and how it might be linked to your own risk? Do you have a family member who has diabetes? Gather this information, record it, and share it with your doctor so together you can make informed decisions about your health. (For a family history tree template, see Appendix D.)

As middle age gets nearer, the 40s is often a decade of rebirth for many women. Some reenter the workforce after raising their children or make a career change, while others have their first baby. Just as these life choices bring about big changes, so can adopting a healthy lifestyle. If habit, denial, and procrastination are slowing you down, remember that you *can* change the less-than-healthy patterns you may have developed in your 20s and 30s, one step at a time. **Resolve to make every calorie count toward good nutrition and every step count toward an active way of life.**

If you've already established healthy eating patterns and an ongoing exercise routine, recommit to keep going and to find ways of accommodating your body's changes that will take you through the years of perimenopause and beyond. In your 40s, your body goes through a phase of significant physical change that rivals puberty, but you have an advantage now that you didn't have as a teenager. You can tune in to your body more effectively and better understand what's happening to it. You are older, but you're also smarter. Use your life skills and insight to manage the process when possible. Embrace the changes and turn this decade into your best so far.

Your heart-health priorities for your 40s are to:

- **Stick to a healthy eating pattern.** Choose a wide variety of foods that provide a high level of nutrition.

- **Stay active.** Make a regular exercise routine part of your daily life so it becomes a lifetime habit. If you need to modify your activities to match your capabilities, experiment to find something you enjoy.

- **Maintain a healthy weight.** Balance your calorie needs with your calorie intake, develop a positive body image, and take pride in taking care of your health. Watch for the triggers that make you vulnerable to weight gain.

- **Know your risks.** If you are at risk, educate yourself and talk with a healthcare professional about what preventive steps are right for you.

- **Develop a good relationship with your doctor.** Get baseline measurements for blood pressure, cholesterol, heart rate, blood glucose, and weight as well as other data you will need to track your health in the future. Talk about how your lifestyle choices may affect your long-term health. If you develop risk factors such as high blood pressure or cholesterol, take action to get them under control and follow the advice of your healthcare providers.

making healthy eating a priority

A healthy diet is the cornerstone of a healthy lifestyle—at any age. Now that you are in your 40s, have you settled into a nutritionally sound eating pattern? Do you eat a varied diet that draws from all the food groups? If not, you're not alone. The demands of family, hectic work schedules, and dieting often contribute to a haphazard approach to good nutrition. There's no changing past eating behaviors, but you have decades ahead to enjoy new, healthy ones. Don't let being busy keep you from tending to your own health needs. Make a commitment to start fresh and develop a healthy eating plan that you can follow for the long term.

Put Nutrition First

A balanced and nourishing eating pattern is a critical part of preventing or delaying many of the conditions that can lead to heart disease. **It's important to evaluate not only the quantity of food you consume but also the quality.** For example, for about the same number of calories, you can eat an average candy bar or a 6-ounce container of fat-free yogurt *and* a medium banana *and* an ounce of low-fat Cheddar cheese and get far more nutritional value for your body. Eat foods that provide nutritional benefits, and focus on "spending" your calories on the foods that give you the best return on your investment. To protect your heart, eat less of the nutrient-poor foods that increase your risk, such as foods high in saturated fat, trans fat, cholesterol, and sodium, and concentrate on unprocessed foods that will meet your nutritional needs and boost your energy and vitality.

Focus on a healthy diet that includes:

- **A variety of vegetables and fruits.** Vegetables and fruits are rich in fiber and offer a wide spectrum of the vitamins and minerals you need to maintain good health. Based on a 2,000-calorie diet, aim for five servings of vegetables and four servings of fruit every day. Easy ways to increase your intake is to add an apple or orange to the small glass of fruit juice you usually have for breakfast, snack on a handful of raisins or dried apricots in the afternoon, and include salads of dark greens and side dishes of carrots or broccoli at lunch and dinner. Research has shown that eating plenty of vegetables and fruits can delay the rise in blood pressure that comes with aging, and in some women it even can help lower high blood pressure levels.

- **Whole-grain and high-fiber foods.** These foods are rich in nutrients, including vitamins, minerals, and fiber. Fiber becomes especially important as the composition of your body begins to change from muscle to fat. Fiber from whole grains can help keep your blood cholesterol levels low or help lower high cholesterol so you can stay off medications longer. In addition to whole-wheat and other whole-grain breads, try whole-grain pastas, brown rice, and lesser-known options such as quinoa. As a rule of thumb, make sure that at least half the grains you eat are whole grains, and try to include about 25 grams of fiber in your diet each day.

- **Fat-free and low-fat dairy products.** The calcium and protein in dairy products are essential in your 40s to keep your bones strong. As you transition into perimenopause, your level of bone-building estrogen starts to decrease. At the same time, your body becomes less able to absorb calcium from food, so you need to take in more. Aim for about 1,000 mg a day, including two to three servings of fat-free or low-fat yogurt, cheeses, milk, and other dairy products or dishes made with them. Low-fat and fat-free cheese cubes make good snacks for the afternoon energy lull, or try a breakfast smoothie of fruit and fat-free milk or yogurt to start your day.

- **Fish rich in omega-3 fatty acids.** Because fish oils are so beneficial for your heart health, try to include at least two servings of fish each week. Tuna, trout, and salmon are high in heart-healthy omega-3 fatty acids, which may decrease levels of LDL cholesterol and triglycerides, lower blood pressure, and reduce the risk of stroke. Omega-3 fats may also fight depression by boosting brain levels of serotonin.

- **Legumes, nuts, and seeds.** Beans, peas, lentils, peanuts, and other members of the legume family are good sources of meatless protein. Making vegetarian meals part of your eating pattern will reduce your intake of the harmful saturated fat found in meats and poultry. Nuts also help maintain healthy blood cholesterol levels because they are rich in heart-healthy unsaturated oils. A small handful of walnuts, almonds, pecans, and most other nuts makes an excellent snack or topping for entrées, salads, and breads. Eat nuts in moderation since they are high in calories.

- **Lean poultry and meats.** Chicken, beef, and pork provide important iron as well as protein. Choose skinless white-meat poultry and lean cuts of meat to keep the saturated fat to a minimum. Aim to eat no more than about 6 ounces of cooked meat or poultry (about 8 ounces raw) a day. A 3-ounce cooked serving should be about the size of a computer mouse or deck of cards.

- **Healthy unsaturated oils and fats.** Replace fats that are high in saturated fat, trans fat, and cholesterol (butter and stick margarine, for example) with unsaturated vegetable oils, such as olive and canola, to help keep down blood cholesterol levels. All fats are high in calories, however, so use them in moderation.

In addition to knowing what foods to include in your diet, it's important to know what to limit. To help you gauge how certain foods fit into your daily eating plan, use these general guidelines as you make your food choices.

- **Aim to limit sodium to less than 2,300 mg each day.** (If you are African American or have high blood pressure, aim for less than 1,500 mg.)

- **Aim to limit cholesterol to less than 300 mg each day.**

- **Aim to limit saturated and trans fats as much as possible.** Try to be sure that your intake of these harmful fats does not reach an unhealthy proportion of your daily calorie intake.

IF YOU USUALLY EAT THIS MANY CALORIES EACH DAY					
	1,200	**1,500**	**1,800**	**2,000**	**2,500**
Keep **saturated fat** to less than	9 grams	11 grams	13 grams	15 grams	19 grams
Keep **trans fat** to less than	1 gram	1.5 gram	2 grams	2 grams	2.5 grams

To revamp your eating habits, start with a quick self-assessment of your current food choices—and be honest with yourself. Do you eat too much junk food or fast food with little nutritional value? Record your current eating habits for a week, writing down *everything* you eat and drink. (See the sample food diary page in Appendix C.) Next to each item, make a note of the meal or time of day and whether anything besides hunger, such as stress or depression, triggered your eating. Look over your week's food log for patterns and evaluate your results. Ask yourself whether you are eating the recommended amounts of vegetables, fruits, and grains each day. Are you eating lots of food high in saturated and trans fats, cholesterol, and sodium? Are you an emotional eater? Decide what you need to cut back on and what you should eat more of, and identify repeated splurges that add up to wasted calories without much nutritional value. Your evaluation may lead to some eye-opening results. If you see patterns that you need to change, plan for alternatives and start new habits that will serve your health better in your 40s.

Here are some ways to boost your nutrition, protect your heart, and keep calories under control in your 40s:

- **Shop smart.** To head off less-than-healthy impulse buying, make a list before you head to the grocery store and stick to it. Avoid shopping on an empty stomach, since hunger makes it harder to resist temptation.

- **Fill your cart first with fresh produce, dairy products, fish, and meats,** all of which usually are located around the perimeter of the store. The packaged and processed foods that tend to be higher in sodium and saturated and trans fats are usually stocked in the inner aisles.

- **Prepare your favorite stews or soups,** then divide them into individual servings and freeze them. Use these easy-to-heat entrées for lunch at work or a busy weekday dinner.

- **Boost your fiber and calcium with vegetables** such as kale, collard greens, napa cabbage, and bok choy. Serve them as side dishes and, depending on the green, add them to salads, soups, stews, or meat loaf for extra nutritional value. Other nondairy sources of calcium include fortified ready-to-eat cereals, sardines, and tofu.

- **Keep washed and cut raw vegetables on hand** for fiber-rich, low-calorie snacking at home and in the office.

- **Take fruit to the office for a quick pick-me-up.** Fruits such as bananas and oranges come naturally "wrapped" and ready to go.

- **Try grilling, broiling, baking, poaching, or pan-searing** different types of fish for healthy and easy meals. Individually wrapped frozen fillets that defrost in 10 minutes are a convenient option for busy weeknight meals.

- Plan to **eat vegetarian meals once or twice a week.** Foods such as edamame or quinoa provide high protein without saturated fat.

- **Eat a whole-grain, high-fiber cereal, such as oatmeal, for breakfast.** Studies have shown that such food can help lower LDL cholesterol.

- **Sprinkle nutrient-packed wheat germ on cereals** or casseroles for crunch and fiber.

- **Prepare homemade snacks,** such as baked tortilla chips made from corn tortillas or trail mix with nuts, high-fiber cereals, and dried fruits.

- **Make snacks ready to go,** by filling small containers or plastic bags with homemade snacks or other portable foods, such as grapes and baby carrots, to grab on your way out the door.

- When you buy packaged snacks, **opt for the ones without saturated or trans fats and with little if any added salt.** Some examples are low-salt pretzels, animal crackers, microwave popcorn, and whole-wheat crackers. Read the nutrition facts panel on labels to find the products lowest in sodium.

- **Boost the magnesium in your diet** with a small handful of almonds or a serving of spinach each day. Magnesium helps regulate your blood pressure and blood sugar levels and plays a role in keeping bones strong.

Because your overall eating pattern is so important to your future health, choose the foods that are best for your body as often as you can.

Focus on making every calorie count toward good nutrition rather than letting convenience or a bad habit dictate your food choices. The fact is that you *can* make a big difference in your long-term heart health by eating wisely now—even if you start with small changes. Those changes will reward you with better nutrition for your body, increased energy and vitality, and improved heart health for the decades ahead.

living an active lifestyle

How do you feel about the E-word ("exercise"?) If you have enjoyed being active most of your life through sports, aerobics classes, or other physical activities, you're likely to think positively about it. However, if you are one of the many women who have not built a routine of physical activity into your lifestyle, the very idea of exercising may make you cringe. In either case, time constraints can make it hard to find a way to fit in fitness in your 40s. Whether your attention has been focused on work, family, or both, **it's time to do something important for yourself** instead of focusing on everyone else.

Let your 40s be the decade that you make being active a top priority. You have many years ahead of you to enjoy the valuable health benefits you can get from adding regular exercise to your life. Make this the time you get moving for a stronger heart.

Why Exercise Is So Important Now

Your metabolism, the chemical process in the body's cells that produces energy from food, slows as you get older, slightly in your 30s and with the real shift occurring in your 40s. With the decline of those energy-producing mechanisms, you require less fuel from the food you eat, and, consequently, as fat gradually replaces muscle mass, subtle changes in your body composition begin. The best way to reenergize, rebuild muscles, and counteract that metabolic shift is to exercise. **Even if you've lapsed into a sedentary lifestyle over the years**—or have never been active at all—**it's not too late to make exercise part of your "prescription" for being and staying healthy.**

Most women's level of physical fitness declines 5 to 10 percent per decade, but it doesn't have to. Regular exercise can slow this decline, and you control how much you exercise each day. A regular routine of aerobic physical activity causes your heart to pump more efficiently, even if you start exercising later in life.

Regular ongoing physical activity will:

- delay the slowing of metabolism

- help you lose or control weight

- lower blood pressure

- reduce harmful LDL cholesterol and increase helpful HDL cholesterol

- reduce the risk of diabetes

- help you develop greater endurance and strength

- strengthen heart muscles and increase cardiovascular capacity

- maintain flexibility

- improve circulation and increase the delivery of oxygen and nutrients to your body's cells

- boost confidence and elevate mood

Regardless of your fitness level, **aerobic conditioning is the best way to strengthen your heart.** Aerobic activities involve moving large muscles, such as those in your legs, with enough intensity to noticeably increase your heart rate (equal to when you walk briskly). A stronger heart muscle and more resilient arteries will allow you to keep exercising at your full capacity as you age and can protect you from heart disease. In addition to exercise that works your cardiovascular system, be sure to include strength training (or resistance training) in your workouts to maintain muscle mass and keep bones strong. Bones are like muscle tissue in that the more you use them, the stronger they get. Weight-bearing exercise, such as climbing stairs, jogging, and participating in sports such as tennis, helps increase bone density as well as your heart rate.

How Much Is Enough?

Being busy is not the same as staying fit. You may believe that you get more exercise than you actually do, especially if you are busy working most of the day. If finding the time is your roadblock, schedule regular physical activity "appointments" the same way you do other commitments.

To assess your activity level, use a pedometer to count the number of steps you take each day. If you take between 5,000 and 7,000, you are a moderately active woman. To be considered very active, you need to log at least 10,000 steps a day. Fewer than about 4,000 is considered inactive.

The recommended **goal for cardiovascular fitness is at least 150 minutes** (2 hours and 30 minutes) **of moderate-intensity or 75 minutes** (1 hour and 15 minutes) **of vigorous-intensity aerobic physical activity each week**—or an equivalent combination of moderate and vigorous activities that will suit your schedule and preferences and meet your goals. Moderate intensity means that you are able to talk during exercise but not sing. Vigorous activities should significantly increase your heart rate, and you should not be able to say more than a few words without catching your breath.

To meet your weekly goal, you could:

- walk at a brisk pace for 35 minutes a day on two days a week, then jog for 20 minutes on two other days.

- spend 30 minutes in a step aerobics class of moderate difficulty five times a week.

- walk briskly for 30 minutes on two days, follow a 60-minute exercise DVD of moderate intensity on one evening, and spend 30 minutes working in your garden (raking, trimming) at a moderate intensity on the weekend.

- work out at the gym on an elliptical machine set to a vigorous-intensity level for 20 minutes on three days, and jog in your neighborhood for 15 minutes on one day.

- walk to and from work fast enough to raise your heart rate, and add 10-minute walks or other aerobic activities during the week to meet the 150-minute recommendation.

Be sure to include strength, or resistance, training at least twice a week to maintain your muscle mass and strengthen bone. Include exercises that involve the major muscle groups of the upper and lower body, in sets of eight to twelve repetitions each.

If you've been sedentary for most of your adult life, the idea of becoming active now may be daunting. It's common to feel a sense of inertia when you're not used to being active, so start with small goals. Consider walking as a possible starting point. It is the easiest way to start a fitness routine—and stick with it—because it is convenient and the only cost is for a pair of good walking shoes. Walking with a friend, spouse, or even your dog increases the likelihood that physical activity will be a regular part of your lifestyle. For starters, take a 10-minute walk at your own pace on at least five days this week, and gradually add another 5 minutes by the end of each successive week. In fact, **short sessions of at least 10 minutes each can add up to the same health benefits as one 30-minute session.** Gradually build up to about 30 minutes total a day, and challenge yourself to walk at a somewhat faster pace each week. A brisk pace (or moderate intensity) is about the same intensity you'd walk if you were late for an important meeting.

If you are an active woman who already enjoys exercise, take a time-out to assess your workout routine and readjust as needed. Even if you've stayed physically active through your 20s and 30s, **you may need to modify your routine and intensity of exercise** to keep in tune with physiological and hormonal changes. Listen to your body. Establish a reasonable regimen that matches your capabilities and doesn't stress your joints. A problematic knee or tennis elbow can keep an otherwise healthy and active 40-something woman on the sidelines for years. Sustaining an injury or dealing with chronic pain can undo your best intentions to stay active.

To stay motivated at any fitness level, set personal goals that are specific and measurable, such as "Starting today, I will go to the gym every other day for two weeks and work out for 30 minutes." **Write down your goals and record your achievements.** (See Appendix C for an activity diary.) Choose a reward that will give you a sense of satisfaction when you reach your goal. Whatever you choose, your real reward will be building the solid foundation for a healthier future.

Make Exercise Enjoyable

When planning how to incorporate exercise into your lifestyle, **be sure to choose physical activities that are fun for you.** By doing so, you'll get a double payoff: exercise and enjoyment, both beneficial to your mental and physical well-being. Even if you are satisfied with your workout routine, consider varying your activities to avoid boredom and burnout. Be creative and try new exercise options. Here are a few suggestions:

- **Exercise with a workout buddy.** Coordinate your schedule with a friend's or coworker's and meet at the gym after work or sign up to take a yoga class together.

- In warmer months, **organize a volleyball game with neighbors** in your backyard. You'll give your heart and lungs a workout while you enjoy the company of others.

- **Go cross-country skiing** (outside or on a machine). The gentle kick and glide technique, combined with the back and forth motion of your arms, provides a better total-body workout than exercise that emphasizes only lower-body muscles.

- **Try water aerobics.** Running, jogging, and walking underwater strengthen leg and hip muscles, develop cardiovascular fitness, and burn calories—without putting stress on your knees and other vulnerable joints.

- **Go swimming.** It helps strengthen the muscles, tendons, and ligaments that support your joints, improving stability and flexibility.

- **Go dancing!** Jazz, ballroom, Latin—even belly— dancing are all fun techniques to get your blood pumping.

- **Kick it up a notch with martial arts,** such as tae kwon do, karate, or kick-boxing; they all develop strength, flexibility, and muscle tone. To get started, work with a qualified instructor so you perform the moves correctly and avoid injury.

- **Take a hike.** Check out online resources to help find trails of varying difficulty in your area. Be sure to wear shoes that provide good ankle support, especially if the trails include rocky terrain.

- **Exercise at work.** If you work in an office, try doing some simple moves at your desk during the day, such as lifting small hand weights or doing pushups against your desk edge while sitting or standing. Also, schedule 10-minute walk breaks on your calendar: one in the morning and one in the afternoon. If you add just two 10-minute breaks every workday, you're two-thirds of the way to reaching the recommended daily goal of 30 minutes!

If you're already physically active, recommit to staying energized and continuing to exercise, even if you need to change your routine to better match your body's capabilities. If you're not active, commit to making a plan to include fitness in your lifestyle and executing it. **You have the power to prevent inactivity from becoming a risk factor for you.** The actions you take now will make a measurable difference in the quality of your life in this decade and those to come.

managing your weight

Like many other 40-something women, you may begin to experience middle-age spread. In fact, **most women gain about 10 pounds in each decade after hitting 40.** That's an extra 20 pounds by age 60! The 40s are such an active time of life—why this tendency toward weight gain?

The hormonal changes of perimenopause coupled with a slowing metabolism tend to make it harder to avoid gaining some additional pounds, especially in the abdomen. During your childbearing years, your body stores fat in areas with estrogen receptors, such as your hips, thighs, and buttocks. Once your estrogen levels start to decline, the receptors aren't activated, and your body begins to store fat in the stomach area instead. The results? A stubborn belly bulge and a thicker waistline. If the number on your scale is inching up, make an action plan to cut back on how much you eat and to add more exercise to your lifestyle. Putting this off for a "better time" is not a good option. If you let extra weight take a firm hold on your body now, you'll have an even harder fight in your 50s because of an increasingly slowing metabolism and menopause.

Another factor that contributes to the tendency to gain weight in your 40s is that you lose muscle with age and thus burn fewer calories each day. For each lost pound of muscle, you burn about 40 fewer calories a day. If the scale shows a gain of 10 pounds after age 40, you probably actually added 15 pounds of fat and lost 5 pounds of muscle. When you notice you're gaining weight, it's a natural reaction to diet, but dramatically cutting back or starving yourself actually can lead to further loss of muscle mass, so you burn even fewer calories.

Being overweight can have many negative consequences, among them the fact that it is a serious risk factor for heart disease. Fortunately, it is a risk factor that you can control. Take that control and commit to losing the extra weight. Reaching and maintaining a healthy weight can be the make-or-break point between ongoing good health and developing health conditions such as high blood pressure, high blood cholesterol, and diabetes. It may also allow you to delay taking heart-related medications for another decade or two. The good news is that losing 10 percent of your body weight—just 10 to 20 pounds for most women—can significantly improve your heart health. The rewards of a more vibrant life as you age will be well worth making the effort now.

Assess Your Eating Habits

Your first step in managing your weight, whether you want to maintain your current weight or drop those extra pounds, is to **determine your body's specific calorie needs and your nutritional needs.** Next, find the right balance between how much you eat and how much you exercise; weight management boils down to a simple equation: calories in = calories out.

To get started, assess your current eating habits by keeping a food and activity diary. For one week, write down everything you eat and drink, with the corresponding calories, and tally the time you spend on physical activity. At the end of the week, add up the calories and divide the total by seven to get your average daily caloric intake. See Appendix C to determine the number of calories you can eat each day to maintain your current weight. If your actual daily calorie intake is more than what you need to maintain your weight, you will gradually gain weight. If you need to lose weight, you will need to find ways to subtract calories from your daily average.

Move More

The best predictor of whether you can avoid excess pounds, or keep off any weight that you lose, is how committed you are to being physically active. An aerobic routine combined with strength training and a healthy diet can burn calories, replace lost muscle, recharge your body's metabolism, and keep extra weight off permanently!

Ideally, to lose weight effectively and keep it off, you may need to aim for 60 to 90 minutes of moderate-intensity aerobic activity every day. If that seems like too much, **start with what's realistic for you.** Sometimes just getting started is the biggest hurdle. A 10-minute walk every day will help you ease into a longer workout routine. Some exercise is always better than no exercise, and every bit of activity adds up to less eventual weight gain.

Try these common-sense approaches to managing your weight in your 40s:

- Make your mantra "**Increase the quality, manage the quantity.**" Choose foods that give you the most nutrition for the calories invested.

- If you need to decrease your calorie intake, **try eating only three-quarters of your usual amount of food.**

- **Find healthier lower-calorie substitutes** you enjoy for foods you eat that are high in calories. For example, if you have a craving for chocolate in the afternoon and end up at the vending machine for a candy bar, try eating a small handful of dark-chocolate-covered raisins instead, saving about 150 calories.

- **Start your meal with a broth-based soup or leafy dark green salad;** either will help fill you up so you will eat less of the meal to follow.

- **Keep portions under control when you eat in restaurants.** Split an entrée or order a couple of appetizers instead of ordering your own entrée. Or, before you start eating, ask for a box to take half your meal home in.

- **Practice eating only when you're hungry.** Listen to your stomach and what it's telling you. Drink some water before you eat. Often you're really more thirsty than hungry.

- **Switch to nutritious snacks** to tide you over between meals. Most nuts, such as almonds and walnuts, provide heart-healthy unsaturated fats, so they make a good choice. Because they are high in calories, though, don't overindulge. A few kinds, such as macadamia nuts and cashews, are high in saturated fats, so eat them sparingly.

- **Don't succumb to your food weaknesses.** Challenge yourself to get creative and find a more healthful solution to satisfy your cravings. Rather than buying ice cream, for example, make your own smoothie with fruit, fat-free yogurt, fat-free milk, and ice. To complete it, add a dollop of fat-free whipped topping, a sprinkling of nuts, and a cherry on top!

- When all you can think of is a certain comfort food, **distract yourself** with something else you enjoy, such as listening to a favorite CD or relaxing in a hot bath. Better yet, walk around the block.

The most effective way to keep your weight under control in your 40s is to find the approach that works best for your lifestyle and your preferences. You may want to drop five pounds as easily as you did in previous decades, but your body isn't as quick to respond as before. You need to accept that with age comes change. Instead of striving for the body you once had, **embrace the body you have now and empower yourself to make it as healthy as you can.** To do that, remember to focus on establishing and maintaining a nutritionally balanced eating plan and finding fun physical activities you enjoy on a regular basis. With these two weapons, you can defend your body from excess pounds, manage your weight throughout your 40s, and avoid the battle of the bulge in your 50s and beyond. Let your 40s be the decade to eat less and move more!

managing your health care

As your body ages during your 40s, it is undergoing subtle physical transitions that leave it more vulnerable, but it is still resilient. **This is a decade when you should monitor your health, listen closely to what your body tells you, and respect the ways in which it is changing.** Although more common in the 50s, conditions such as high blood pressure or high cholesterol may start to appear in your 40s. If you keep a watchful eye on your baseline health measurements, you'll be aware early of any developing changes and be able to take action to manage them effectively.

Establish Your Healthcare Team

A comfortable working partnership with doctors you trust should be at the core of your health care. If you haven't teamed up with healthcare professionals with whom you can talk openly and whom you trust to look out for your best interests, make it your priority to do so. Assemble a good team of healthcare professionals now so they'll be in place *before* you have a serious health concern.

To increase the likelihood that developing risk factors or disease symptoms will be identified and managed as early as possible, be sure to set up annual physical checkups. (To learn which tests are age appropriate and should be included in your annual healthcare visits, see Appendix A.) Get your test results in writing or write them down yourself. You'll be more active in managing your health if you set up your own system for recording your results using your home computer, an online program, or a health diary. Getting annual checkups and keeping good health records are both important ways to take an active role in managing your health care.

Once you establish your healthcare team, probably a general practitioner or internist and an ob-gyn, share your medical information with them. **You are the critical link in the communication about your**

health, so be an active participant in the management of your own health care. If you are concerned about a new symptom or have a question, don't hesitate to share that concern with your healthcare providers. Each piece of information—even if you think it may not be important or aren't sure how it might connect with the rest—can be a vital clue to a more accurate diagnosis or helpful lifestyle recommendation. Also, let your healthcare providers know what, if any, medications you are taking, including prescriptions, over-the-counter meds, vitamins, and herbal products. (For additional information on communicating with your healthcare providers, see Appendix B.)

Managing Risk Factors in Your 40s

While you are in your 40s, you and your healthcare team need to assess all the heart disease risk factors you may be facing. Perimenopause brings with it many physiological changes that put your heart at greater risk. Changes in hormone levels coincide with increased weight gain and higher blood pressure and cholesterol, for example. Now is the time to decide what you can do to work toward a healthier heart if you have any of the following risk factors.

If your healthcare providers diagnose a developing risk factor when you are in your 40s, you are benefiting from advances in early detection and treatment that are now available. Medical research focused specifically on women's heart health has brought about a shift in how doctors view their younger female patients and their risk of disease. For years, the hormone estrogen was thought to protect premenopausal women from heart disease, so heart disease was not considered a real threat until after menopause. As science has shown, however, the risk factors that lead to heart disease start much earlier; consequently, more emphasis is being placed on prevention of heart disease in younger women.

FAMILY HISTORY
Take the time in your 40s to be sure your family medical history information is up to date. If you haven't shared this information with your healthcare providers, be sure to do so, or update any changes if your family history is already in your health records. Some risk factors for heart disease are hereditary and could begin to surface in your 40s, so if you are at risk, be especially vigilant.

HIGH BLOOD PRESSURE

Because of the effects of age and typical lifestyle habits, your blood pressure may start to rise in your 40s. In fact, almost one-third of women have high blood pressure by age 55. If your blood pressure measures over 120/80 mmHg but under 140/90 on more than two occasions, your doctor may diagnose you as having *prehypertension*. That designation means that your blood pressure levels are on the border between healthy and dangerous. Because of increased awareness of the destructive effects of untreated high blood pressure, the cutoff point for what is considered a harmful level of blood pressure has been lowered, and the category of prehypertension was established to call attention to the condition sooner. As a result, doctors are more careful than ever to aggressively treat prehypertension before it progresses into full-blown high blood pressure (140/90 mmHg or higher).

If you are black and in your 40s, be sure to have your blood pressure checked often. African American women are even more susceptible to high blood pressure than whites, and at an earlier age as well. Also, especially if you're black or Hispanic, be aware of any sudden changes in your ability to exercise, such as getting tired or out of breath sooner than usual. Studies have shown that these changes can be a sign of heart disease in women, so don't be reluctant to tell your doctor, even if you think it will turn out to be a false alarm.

If you are prehypertensive or have high blood pressure, work with your healthcare providers to get your blood pressure under control. You can help lower your blood pressure by eating a healthy diet, exercising regularly, and losing weight if necessary. It's also important to quit smoking and limit your alcohol intake.

HIGH CHOLESTEROL AND TRIGLYCERIDES

Before the onset of menopause, you do have some natural protection against heart disease, which is reflected in your lipid profile (the levels of LDL cholesterol, HDL cholesterol, triglycerides, and other fats that are measured in your blood). As you go through perimenopause, fluctuations in hormone levels can result in an increase in harmful LDL and triglycerides, and a simultaneous decrease in helpful HDL cholesterol. Now is the time for you and your doctor to monitor your blood lipids for changes that signal potential developing problems.

american heart association
complete guide to women's heart health

OBESITY AND PHYSICAL INACTIVITY

Weight gain, another effect of perimenopause, and a general decrease in the level of physical activity that many women experience in their 40s are separate but often interrelated risk factors for heart disease. In particular, the amount of visceral fat, or belly fat, that accumulates around your waist is a good indicator of how much at risk you are. If your waist measures 35 inches or more, you should lose weight to reduce your risk. **Being inactive by itself increases the tendency to gain weight and is linked with higher blood pressure, higher LDL cholesterol levels, and a greater likelihood of developing diabetes.** You can lessen these risks with a regular program of moderate physical activity.

DIABETES

Diabetes is a major risk factor for heart disease if left unmanaged, particularly in women. Its development is linked to obesity, changes in metabolism, and a sedentary lifestyle. Type 2 diabetes, by far the most common kind, develops gradually as your body begins to respond to insulin less and less efficiently (known as insulin resistance). **Type 2 diabetes is most commonly seen after age 45,** but the incidence in younger women is increasing. African American, Hispanic, and Native American women are at higher risk for diabetes and are more likely to develop it at a younger age. Because you can have diabetes without knowing it, you should have a fasting blood glucose test every three years after age 45. Diabetes is defined as a fasting blood glucose reading of 126 mg/dL or more, and the condition called insulin resistance or prediabetes is defined as a reading between 100 and 125 mg/dL. If your blood glucose level is higher than normal, your first steps in managing the progression of diabetes are to eat a

Pregnancy can bring on certain changes in your circulatory system, such as change in blood pressure and blood circulation, and other conditions that can affect your heart health (see page 65). If you're pregnant or thinking of becoming pregnant, talk with your doctor about your heart-related risk factors. If you were diagnosed with gestational diabetes when pregnant, you are at higher risk for developing diabetes now. Be sure that your healthcare provider checks your fasting blood sugar yearly so you can detect changes that indicate prediabetes or type 2 diabetes. If your blood pressure became elevated during pregnancy, your risk of developing high blood pressure after pregnancy is also significantly increased.

balanced diet, exercise regularly, lose weight, and monitor your blood glucose carefully. If you already have diabetes, work with your healthcare providers to keep it under control.

METABOLIC SYNDROME

Having one risk factor for heart disease increases your risk, but having more than one increases it significantly. If you have a combination of several risk factors, you have metabolic syndrome, which puts you at higher risk for heart attack after menopause. These are the signals your healthcare providers look for to identify metabolic syndrome:

- Waist measurement equal to or greater than 35 inches

- Triglyceride level of 150 mg/dL or higher

- HDL cholesterol less than 50 mg/dL

- Systolic blood pressure of 130 mmHg or higher

- Diastolic blood pressure of 85 mmHg or higher

- Fasting glucose reading of 100 mg/dL or higher

If you have metabolic syndrome, controlling one or all of these risk factors with a balanced heart-healthy diet, a regular exercise routine (preferably vigorous intensity), and weight loss will greatly reduce your risk for heart disease.

BIRTH CONTROL/HORMONE THERAPY

If you are taking birth control pills or thinking of adding hormone replacement therapy in your 40s, you should carefully consider the risks and benefits for your personal situation. Talk with your doctor, gather as much information as you can, and make an informed decision that suits your healthcare needs best. Low-dose oral contraceptives don't increase your risk of heart attack unless they are combined with other risk factors, such as smoking, high blood pressure, or high cholesterol. However, as you enter perimenopause, it's more likely that you will develop high blood pressure or high cholesterol. (If you've had surgically induced menopause, that too needs to be factored into your healthcare equation and subsequent decisions.) Because of the risks associated with hormone replacement therapy (including increased risk of cardiovascular events and breast cancer), it should be used only when needed to relieve the symptoms of perimenopause, not as a means to restore skin tone or delay other normal signs of aging. (For more information on hormone therapy, see page 121.)

POLYCYSTIC OVARY SYNDROME

This is a common disorder of the endocrine system that disrupts a woman's normal hormonal cycles. It's usually identified in women who have trouble conceiving in their 30s. Symptoms include obesity, increased waist measurement, insulin resistance, high blood pressure, higher levels of LDL cholesterol, and lower levels of HDL cholesterol—all of which increase the risk of heart disease. If you've been diagnosed with this condition, be proactive in your 40s by carefully monitoring your risk factors, eating a healthy diet, and being physically active on a regular basis.

• • •

You can prepare for the physical changes of perimenopause by making a personal commitment to play an active role in your risk factor management. Take control of your heart health by working with your healthcare team to identify your own personal risk factors and determine how best to manage them. **Continue to take *preventive* steps to reduce your risks** by eating for good nutrition, participating in a regular fitness routine, managing your weight, and getting annual checkups—all important actions that will make a measurable difference in your overall heart health. These things take a time commitment on your part, and you probably lead a busy, busy life. However, by being proactive in your 40s, you can protect your heart health *before* heart disease has a chance to sneak up on you.

checklist for achieving heart health in your 40s

✓ **Make it a priority to get healthier,** especially if you plan to have children.

✓ **Learn to make every calorie count** for good nutrition.

✓ **Establish a plan to make** healthy eating and regular exercise part of your regular routine.

✓ **Follow the plan** and modify it if necessary.

✓ Fight a tendency to gain weight by **cutting back a little on calories** and being physically active to keep your weight at a healthy level.

✓ **Establish and maintain working relationships with trusted healthcare professionals.**

✓ **Get regular health checkups** and know your numbers.

✓ **Be aware of and manage your risk factors**—especially smoking, elevated blood pressure, diabetes, and overweight and obesity.

Hormone Therapy: What Is Right for You?

Postmenopausal hormone therapy, formerly known as hormone replacement therapy or HRT, has become a confusing, even frightening, issue for many women. If you are going through perimenopause or menopause, you may be trying to sort out the risks and benefits of using hormones. Knowing how hormone therapy evolved and how it has been perceived in the past may help you make a more informed decision about what is best for you.

As a woman goes through perimenopause, her levels of the hormones estrogen and progesterone fluctuate until they flatten out at true menopause—defined as 12 months after the last period. With the hormonal fluctuations come symptoms such as hot flashes, mood swings, sleeplessness, and vaginal dryness or discomfort, among others. For years, healthcare providers prescribed artificial hormones (commonly estrogen plus progestin, which is synthetic progesterone) to ease the discomfort of these symptoms.

At the same time, it was hoped that restoring premenopausal hormone levels would also restore the protection against cardiovascular disease that women seem to have before menopause. (Based on the observation that most women do not show signs of heart disease until well after menopause, researchers theorized that female hormones estrogen and progesterone offered natural protection. Therefore, if the missing hormones were replaced, a postmenopausal woman would regain the same degree of protection.)

For years it was widely believed that hormone therapy would help alleviate menopausal symptoms, ward off heart disease and osteoporosis, improve skin and hair tone, and generally keep women young—but **researchers now know that hormone therapy is not the magic formula they hoped for.** The Women's Health Initiative (WHI) study, which had set out to assess both the benefits and risks of hormone therapy, was stopped prematurely in 2002 because of findings that indicated more health risk than benefit in the women taking hormone therapy. It appeared that the trial combination of estrogen and

continued

progestin was associated with an increased risk of breast cancer but not with cardiovascular benefit. And surprisingly, the study also found that **hormone therapy was associated with a higher risk of coronary artery disease, heart attack, stroke, and blood clots.**

This information led to a significant change in thinking regarding the use of hormone therapy. Women and healthcare providers alike became more wary of the risks, and many women stopped using hormones altogether. Since 2002, however, more recent studies suggest that the cardiovascular risk may not be as significant for younger women who use hormone therapy to manage the symptoms of menopause, as opposed to women who used hormone therapy later in life to protect against heart disease. Research is continuing to determine how hormone therapy affects the development of heart disease and whether there is a "time window" in which it may be most useful.

Based on the current research, **the American Heart Association does not advise women to use postmenopausal hormone therapy or selective estrogen receptor modulators to reduce the risk of coronary artery disease or stroke.** If your symptoms of menopause are severe enough to disrupt your well-being, you should **discuss both the risks and benefits in your individual situation with your healthcare professional.** Hormone therapy has both positive and negative effects on your body, and every woman's needs are different. If you do not experience troublesome menopausal symptoms, you do not need hormone therapy, and you should not use it if you have heart disease, breast cancer, or a history of blood clots.

If you *do* decide to use hormone therapy, the best approach is to take the lowest effective dose for the shortest time possible and to periodically reassess the risk-versus-benefit equation for your own situation. Try to use the delivery method that best addresses your symptoms with the lowest dosage: estrogen is available in a pill, patch, gel, or vaginal cream. If you are taking HRT at the moment and are planning to stop, expect some symptoms to return, no matter what your age, but you can work with your healthcare provider to create a step-down plan that minimizes discomfort.

CHAPTER 6

your 50s

. . .

After watching my father, mother, and friends battle heart disease, I'm determined to reduce my risk. For the first time, I'm paying attention to the cholesterol and blood pressure numbers my doctor gives me. Now I know my numbers. I know that my heart health is in my hands. —DEBBIE, 58

. . .

If you're in your 50s, you're probably in transition.

Perhaps you're reentering the workforce or thinking of changing careers. Maybe you're an empty nester who finally has time to explore new interests and reinvent your social life. One thing is certain—**your body is changing and those changes affect your heart.**

Menopause brings with it an increased risk for heart disease. If you've made it to your 50s without developing the major risk factors for heart disease, keep up the good work. If, like many other 50-something women, you are facing risk factors such as high cholesterol or elevated blood pressure, make the most of this time of transition to control or reduce them. Healthy eating habits and increased physical activity can still have a profoundly positive effect on your long-term health.

Use the life management skills you've acquired to take better care of yourself:

- **Make every calorie count.** Most women gain a few pounds after menopause, so be watchful that the pounds don't keep escalating.

- **Get or stay physically active.** Find an activity you enjoy that gets you moving on a regular basis. Since you start to lose muscle mass as you age, exercise is vital to your overall well-being.

- **Make sure your heart health is part of every physical exam.** You and your doctor should be tracking your weight, blood pressure, cholesterol levels, and heart rate.

Make healthy lifestyle choices now to increase your odds for a long and vital life.

introduction

Many women find their 50s to be the best years of their lives. The combination of significant life achievements tempered by life experience makes most women at this age confident, focused, and well equipped to cope with life, both the day-to-day misadventures and the major challenges. Yet with this sense of sureness and centeredness comes the bittersweet reality of aging.

Even if you are among the fittest and most disciplined of women, you'll begin to see some physical signs of aging in your 50s. The loss of muscle tone may cause your face to soften, and a slowing metabolism may lead to a thickening waist, even though your weight hasn't increased. What you *can't* see as you age is that your heart is physically changing as well, and so is the complex cardiovascular system that supports it. It's these changes that increase your risk for heart disease.

Although the risk for heart disease is real, it's important to realize that you can proactively limit that risk. **Your lifestyle choices, particularly those involving smoking, nutrition, physical activity, and** weight management, can still have a huge impact on your heart. And there's a bonus: many of the things you do to improve and maintain your heart health also can improve your mood, energy level, and mental well-being, making you feel better and younger.

Statistics show that in terms of risk, women lag behind men by about 10 years; nevertheless, the risk for women—especially women over 50— is real. **If you are a woman in your 50s,** you therefore need to be aware that **you have moved into a new risk group for heart disease and heart attack.** The number of women who have heart attacks escalates dramatically after age 55. In fact, **cardiovascular disease is the leading cause of death in women—especially after menopause.**

But that doesn't mean you should give up and give in. Heart disease is not an inevitable part of getting older, and if you do find you have a form of heart disease, you can do a lot to help manage it. Now is the time to focus your lifetime of organizational and management skills on your own health.

Understanding How Your Body Is Changing

Aging is, of course, a gradual process. It actually starts during your 20s, but when you are in your 50s, you are more likely to notice its effects on your body. As you get older, your heart and other organs undergo changes in structure and function. Gradually your heart becomes slightly enlarged, and the chamber walls thicken. Also, your arteries slowly stiffen and become less elastic, so they cannot contract and relax as quickly as they used to. In fact, a recent study found that this increased arterial stiffness appears to coincide with menopause. Over time, all these changes will affect your heart's ability to pump blood efficiently and deliver oxygen and nutrients to your body's cells. For an overview of the gradual physiological changes in the aging heart, see page 184.

You may not realize it, but now that you are in your 50s, chances are your arteries have a lining of plaque that has accumulated throughout your lifetime. That plaque can lead to heart disease and heart attack. The influence of genetics and your previous and current lifestyle choices are now coming into play too. When you combine these with the effects of menopause, your body becomes increasingly vulnerable to heart disease.

| american heart association
complete guide to women's heart health

For most women, actual menopause occurs around the age of 50, after the years of gradual transformation called perimenopause. **Menopause itself does not cause heart disease,** but the loss of natural hormones such as estrogen after menopause may contribute to increases in harmful LDL cholesterol and triglycerides, decreases in helpful HDL cholesterol, and alterations in the walls of blood vessels—all physical changes that do put you at higher risk. You may find that, for the first time in your life, you need to take prescription drugs to manage risk factors such as high blood pressure or elevated cholesterol levels, or you may begin to put on abdominal weight that wasn't a problem in your 30s or 40s. You may need to adjust your lifestyle as your body changes.

Making Your Health a Top Priority

Some women in their 50s lament "getting old," so they begin to think about "fixes," such as having cosmetic surgery for sagging eyelids or liposuction for that stubborn belly fat—personal choices related to *looking* older. But now is the time to deal constructively with *feeling* older. The lifestyle choices you make today in your 50s can help you feel stronger, be more energetic, and maintain vitality in the decades to come.

Growing evidence shows that by adopting healthy lifestyle habits, **you can slow down or even stop the progression of risk factors that threaten your heart.** Some researchers believe that **you even may be able to undo damage from your earlier years by breaking unhealthy habits.** Thanks to this increased awareness of the importance of lifestyle choices, you have the opportunity to learn how you can protect your heart and reduce your chance of dying of heart disease. As a woman who has experience in making choices, you can choose to take advantage of the newest research and manage your health in a smart way.

Think about your health the way you think about your finances: just as you might review your investments with your financial planner to see whether you have a healthy portfolio, you and your healthcare professionals should evaluate your physical well-being for a heart-healthy future. **Eating a healthy diet, developing and executing a plan for regular physical activity, controlling your weight, and managing your** other risk factors—all are your best defenses against heart disease and heart attack.

Your heart-health priorities for your 50s are to:

- **Establish a nutritious eating plan.** Eat a variety of foods from all food groups and determine your personal caloric needs.

- **Be physically active.** Regular exercise is a key element to keeping your heart strong. Find some physical activity that you enjoy doing and stick with it.

- **Maintain a healthy weight.** It's not too late to establish a healthy weight and learn how to maintain it. Although the bikinis and tight jeans of former decades may be long gone, there are still enormous long-term heart-health benefits to achieving and sustaining a healthy weight.

- **Monitor your existing risk factors.** Be aware of *all* your risk factors for heart disease, but pay special attention to those that may be increasing because of age and menopause, such as elevated blood pressure and higher levels of cholesterol.

- **Manage the risk factors that you *can* control or change.** Eating well and exercising regularly are important actions that you can take to limit your risk for heart disease. Accept and make peace with those things you cannot change.

- **Recruit a team of healthcare providers.** Find doctors you trust to monitor and manage risk factors *before* you have any serious health issues.

- **Take your medications to control risk factors.** If medications for high blood pressure, high cholesterol, diabetes, or other heart-health risks have been prescribed, be sure to take them as directed by your healthcare provider.

- **Educate yourself about any heart condition you may have.** Partner with your healthcare providers and ask questions until you fully understand the treatment options open to you and can take advantage of recent medical advances.

american heart association
complete guide to women's heart health

making healthy eating a priority

By the time you've reached your 50s, some of your previous lifestyle choices, especially poor eating habits, are probably taking a toll on your health, but it's not too late to start eating well now. Researchers who have studied how lifestyle changes affect heart health found that **women who switched to a heart-healthy diet and increased their amount of exercise slowed the buildup of plaque in their arteries.** Not only is embracing a healthy diet good for your heart, it also increases your energy level and boosts your overall vitality.

Healthy Food, Healthy Body

It's now more important than ever to focus on incorporating nutritious foods—the ones that offer the best health payoff—into your overall eating pattern. The return on your investment in healthy eating is twofold: it increases your heart-health assets with a good balance of important nutrients, and it decreases heart-health liabilities such as high LDL cholesterol and high blood pressure levels. To help control your risk for heart disease, you need to **eat more nutrient-dense foods,** such as vegetables, fruits, and whole grains, and fewer of the foods that contain saturated fat, trans fat, cholesterol, and sodium—all nutritional foes that often come from packaged convenience foods and fast foods.

A healthy diet includes:

- **A variety of colorful vegetables and fruits.** The more variety you fit into your diet, the wider the range of nutrients—vitamins, minerals, and fiber—with which you will reward your body. Choose the vegetables and fruits that are deepest in color; the deeper the color, the higher the level of nutrients. Based on a 2,000-calorie diet, aim for about five servings of vegetables and four servings of fruit each day.

- **Whole-grain and high-fiber foods.** Like deeply colored fruits and vegetables, these foods provide essential vitamins, minerals, and fiber. Fiber plays an important role in heart health by helping lower harmful LDL cholesterol levels. Good sources of whole grains include whole-wheat breads, whole-wheat pasta, brown rice, and whole-grain cereal. At least half your grain servings should be whole grains, so check the labels on grain products to be sure a *whole* grain is the first ingredient. Other high-fiber foods include beans, fruits, and vegetables. Aim to include at least 21 grams of fiber each day in your diet. Some easy ways to add fiber to your diet are by eating whole-grain cereal for breakfast, adding beans or other legumes to a salad with lunch or dinner, and eating whole fruits and vegetables, including the peels, throughout the day.

- **Fish rich in omega-3 fatty acids.** Studies have shown that omega-3 fatty acids in the diet reduce the risk of coronary artery disease. Make it a goal to eat fatty fish, such as salmon, tuna, and trout, at least twice a week. If you have heart disease or high triglycerides, check with your healthcare provider about taking omega-3 supplements as well.

- **Fat-free and low-fat dairy products.** Women need adequate calcium throughout their lives, but after menopause it's even more important in order to prevent the onset of osteoporosis and other bone conditions. You should consume two to three servings of fat-free or low-fat dairy products a day. An 8-ounce container of fat-free or low-fat yogurt contains about 450 mg of calcium, nearly half the daily recommendation. Vegetable greens, as well as some soybean products and other legumes, also provide calcium. For example, a cup of kale contains 90 mg of calcium. The daily recommendation for women over 50 is 1,200 mg, but ask your healthcare provider how much is right for you.

- **Lean poultry and meats.** If you'd like to include poultry and meat in your diet, do it! Just keep two small portions a day (each about 3 ounces cooked, or the size of your computer mouse or a deck of cards), choose lean skinless poultry, such as white-meat chicken and turkey, and lean cuts of meat, such as eye-of-round roast and sirloin steak, and remove all the visible fat.

american heart association
complete guide to women's heart health

- **Legumes, nuts, and seeds.** Legumes, such as peas, peanuts and peanut butter, beans, and lentils, are great sources of fiber and meatless protein. Nuts and seeds are rich in helpful monounsaturated fats, and when they are part of a diet that also is low in saturated fat and cholesterol they may actually help keep down blood cholesterol levels.

- **Healthy unsaturated oils and fats.** As often as you can, replace harmful fats that are high in saturated fat, trans fat, and cholesterol (typically animal fats such as butter and hydrogenated stick margarine) with unsaturated vegetable oils, such as olive and canola. Including these healthier fats will help keep blood cholesterol levels low and reduce the progression of atherosclerosis. Because all fats are high in calories, use them in moderation.

In addition to knowing what foods to include in your diet, it's important to know what to limit. To help you gauge how certain foods fit into your eating plan, use these guidelines as you make your food choices.

- **Aim to limit sodium to less than 1,500 mg a day.** Middle-aged women, especially African Americans and women with high blood pressure, need less than the 2,300 mg recommended for healthy younger adults.

- **Aim to limit cholesterol to less than 300 mg each day.**

- **Aim to limit saturated and trans fats as much as possible.** Try to be sure that your intake of these harmful fats does not reach an unhealthy proportion of your daily calorie intake.

IF YOU USUALLY EAT THIS MANY CALORIES EACH DAY					
	1,200	1,500	1,800	2,000	2,500
Keep **saturated fat** to less than	9 grams	11 grams	13 grams	15 grams	19 grams
Keep **trans fat** to less than	1 gram	1.5 gram	2 grams	2 grams	2.5 grams

As you develop your eating plan, be sure to include a variety of healthy choices from all these food groups so you don't feel deprived and to ensure that you get maximum, balanced nutritional value. A potassium-rich diet, for example, is essential in regulating blood pressure, yet many women need to increase their potassium intake. Potassium-rich foods include bananas, orange juice, sweet potatoes, fat-free and low-fat yogurt, spinach, and tomatoes. Aim for 4,700 mg of potassium a day, but check with your healthcare provider about what's right for you since too much potassium can be as harmful as too little. Eating foods that provide calcium and vitamin D helps prevent bone loss after 50. Good sources of calcium include fat-free and low-fat dairy products. Foods that provide vitamin D include fat-free and low-fat milk, salmon, mackerel, sardines, and some fortified cereals. Adequate sun exposure is also important in getting sufficient vitamin D. Another nutrient often lacking in women's diets is magnesium. Good sources of magnesium are whole-grain foods, green leafy vegetables, nuts, and dried peas and beans.

Plan Well, Eat Well

Following a heart-healthy diet takes both discipline and good planning, but the payoff is worth the investment. Without planning, it's easier to grab a fast-food meal when you're on the run and to give in to those high-calorie, high-fat treats for a grab-and-go snack. It's important to make every calorie count, however. Good nutrition always trumps convenience!

Now that you are in your 50s, you may be regaining some control of your time. If your children are more independent these days, perhaps you can turn the attention you once paid to packing school lunches and preparing kid-friendly meals back to yourself. You can replace the tendency to grab meals helter-skelter because of hectic family schedules with a more thoughtful, healthy approach to meal planning. If you have children at home, designate certain nights as family nights and enjoy a healthy home-cooked meal together. Conversely, if you and your partner are now empty nesters or if you are single and haven't already been doing so, perhaps it's time to make cooking healthy at home part of your regular weekly routine. Whatever your situation, **make it a priority in your 50s to establish heart-healthy eating patterns.**

To get started, record your current eating habits for a week, writing down *everything* you eat and drink. We've included a sample food diary page at the end of Appendix C. Beside each item, make a note of the meal or time of day and whether you ate because of anything besides hunger, such as stress or depression. At the end of a week's time, conduct a quick self-assessment of your current eating plan—and be honest with yourself. Are you eating the foods that provide you with the best health payoff? Do you eat too much junk food or fast food with little nutritional value that is high in saturated and trans fats, cholesterol, and sodium? Are you eating too much food? Are you an emotional eater?

Your evaluation may lead to some interesting discoveries. Look for patterns and evaluate your results. Try to find ways to be sure you get the recommended amounts of vegetables, fruits, and grains each day. Decide where you need to cut back, and what foods you should eat more of. Maybe you need to make only small modifications to eat better—or maybe you need an extreme nutrition makeover. Wherever on the spectrum you fall, you can make the changes needed to move—or continue to move—in the direction of healthy eating. Just as you likely have revised your wardrobe, makeup, and hairstyle in your 50s to best complement how you look on the outside, it's also time to change your eating habits to better match your needs on the *inside*.

Here are some easy tips for healthy eating:

- **Start thinking of meat as a side dish** so that you have room to add more vegetables, fruits, and grains to your meals.

- **Think of fresh fruit as the ultimate convenience food**—it comes in its own packaging and can easily go almost anywhere with you.

- **Prepare your favorite vegetables**—either raw or cooked—and take small snack packs to work to munch on when hunger strikes or to complement a frozen-entrée lunch.

- **Make a batch of broth-based vegetable soup and freeze it** in individual containers so it's easily available, quick to defrost, and single-serving ready. A cup of soup before meals will give you additional servings of vegetables and fiber and make you feel fuller. Soup also makes a satisfying mid-afternoon snack at work to replace the vending machine candy bar.

- **Keep a bag of prewashed spinach in the refrigerator.** Add it to lots of dishes—soups, spaghetti sauces, casseroles, vegetable dips—in addition to salads, of course. Spinach provides lots of dark green goodness, including fiber and iron.

- **Eat 1½ ounces, or a small handful, of nuts**—such as almonds or walnuts—four or five days a week. Nuts are rich in the good unsaturated oils and can help satisfy hunger, but they are high in calories so keep portions small.

- **Be creative with your salads**—experiment by adding fruits, nuts, or unfamiliar vegetables to your favorite mix of greens.

- **Add fish to your diet** by purchasing salmon or low-sodium tuna in cans or pouches and enjoying it in a salad or whole-wheat pita for lunch. Make fish your go-to meal when you eat out to add servings of omega-3 to your diet.

- **Use edamame** (green soybeans) **for an all-purpose protein and fiber boost** in salads, entrées, and snacks—or eat it just by itself!

- **Replace the usual white breads, pasta, and rice with their whole-grain versions.**

- **Be a label detective** in the grocery store and investigate ways to avoid high-sodium processed foods.

The nutritional stakes get higher with each decade, and the bottom line is that in your 50s you have to pay more attention to what you eat than you did in your 30s and 40s. It's okay to splurge once in a while; the overall pattern of how you choose to eat is what counts. You can still eat delicious food and enjoy it, but learn to choose your foods wisely.

living an active lifestyle

If you're in your 50s, you already know you have to work with your body's physical changes to stay fit. Being active now will be easier if you have made exercise part of your routine all along. But if you've been sedentary for most of your life, the idea of making a major lifestyle switch to more physical activity can be overwhelming. It's not hard to find reasons not to exercise: no time, no energy, no motivation—whatever the excuses, they are obstacles to good health and they need to be overcome. Why? Because by the time you reach your 50s, **you *must* be physically active on a regular basis for the sake of your heart health.**

Why Exercise Is So Important to Your Heart

Being physically active is important at any age: studies show that **improved fitness results in a longer life of greater quality.** Once you reach your 50s, however, exercise becomes an essential component of good health in your future. You are at a turning point because you're dealing with the physiological changes of menopause that make you vulnerable to heart disease. If exercise is part of your lifestyle, you will have a powerful tool on your side to help counteract the effects of age and menopause, increase your vitality, and protect your heart.

Aerobic exercise uses large muscle groups to increase your heart rate. For the greatest health benefit, you'll want to combine aerobic conditioning with some kind of strength or resistance training and weight-bearing exercise to maintain your muscle mass and strengthen your bones. **An ongoing routine of regular moderately intense or vigorous physical activity will:**

- balance a slower metabolism

- help you lose or control weight

- reduce arterial stiffening

- lower blood pressure

- reduce harmful LDL cholesterol and increase helpful HDL cholesterol

- reduce the risk of diabetes

- slow the rate of bone loss that occurs after menopause

- help you develop greater endurance and strength

- strengthen heart muscle and increase cardiovascular capacity

- maintain flexibility

- improve circulation and increase the delivery of oxygen and nutrients to your body's cells

- boost confidence and elevate mood

Taking the "In" Out of "Inactivity"

Just as there are benefits to being physically active, there are consequences for being *in*active. **Inactivity is largely responsible for much of the physical decline considered a "normal" part of the aging process.** Being sedentary is so detrimental to good health that it is now classified as a major risk factor for heart disease and stroke as well as for many other health problems.

Never exercised before? Think you're too old? Have physical conditions that need to be considered? Don't let any of that stop you. Don't give in to the idea that exercise won't help or will be too hard. **If exercise is new to you, begin slowly.** Physical activity doesn't need to be an all-or-nothing proposition. You don't need to start marathon training, but you could try walking around your local high school track or in a nearby mall. Start off with just a 10-minute walk and work up to a daily 30-minute walk. Even if you start slowly, you can do a lot to improve your heart health. Keep in mind that **doing *something* is better than doing nothing.** (Use the activity diary in Appendix C to record your progress.)

But what if you were always fairly fit and now find it physically difficult to continue the activities you once enjoyed? Try creatively changing your routine to allow for physical limitations you may now have. If you were a runner when you were younger, switch to brisk walking or water aerobics for less stress on your knees and ankles. If you loved ballet, try a similar discipline that also focuses on a strong center, such as Pilates or yoga. Just be mindful to **take care of your joints and listen to your body.** Routine weight-bearing exercise, such as working with weights or walking, builds up muscle mass that helps protect against injury.

Finding Fun in Fitness at Any Level

First and foremost, find a physical activity that you already like to do or are interested in trying. Studies show that if you enjoy the activity, you will stick with it.

Here are some tips on how to add physical activity into your lifestyle:

- **Think of ways to combine your hobbies or interests with a physical activity.** If you're a nature lover, photographer, or bird-watcher, for example, go to local walking paths or hiking trails, take a 30-minute walk, and spend some time before or after to enjoy your hobby.

- **Turn physical activity into a social experience.** Join a gym or your town's community activity center, participate in local charity walks, take yoga or ballroom dancing, or walk with friends, neighbors, or family members. You're more likely to stick to an activity if others are involved with you.

- If you prefer some solitude or quiet time, **try an early morning walk with your dog or take a walk around your office** or at a nearby mall at lunchtime to give yourself a break from work. When you exercise alone, you can calm your mind and let it drift to thoughts you enjoy.

- **Incorporate more physical activity in atypical ways.** For example, set up a regular date night with your significant other or a friend. Be adventurous and bring out that inner kid in you. Skip the movies and instead try bowling, dancing, or whatever you enjoy together that gets you up and moving.

- **Wear a pedometer and record how many steps you take each day** for a week. Use the average as a baseline and try to add 250 or more steps each day. For example, walk around the perimeter of the grocery store a few times when you go shopping or walk around your office building before you go home. Simple little routines can add up to a lot of steps. Your ultimate goal is to aim for 10,000 steps each day.

How Much Is Enough?

Whatever aerobic activity you choose, **your goal should be at least 150 minutes** (2 hours and 30 minutes) **of moderate-intensity aerobic exercise a week, or 75 minutes** (1 hour and 15 minutes) **of more vigorous intensity,** or an equivalent combination of moderate and vigorous to suit your schedule and preference. "Moderate intensity" means that as you are exercising, you notice that your heart rate increases but you can still talk. "Vigorous" means that the activity level should make you breathe rapidly and substantially increase your heart rate; you can say only a few words without stopping to catch your breath.

You could reach these goals each week by including 30 minutes of vigorous aerobic dancing twice a week and 60 minutes of ballroom dancing (moderate intensity) once a week, and taking a 30-minute brisk walk once. Aerobic activity should be performed in episodes of at least 10 minutes, and preferably spread out through the week.

If you don't have the time to participate in a physical activity for 30 minutes at one time, just walk briskly (or enjoy some other moderately intense activity) for 10 minutes two or three times a day; the benefits are cumulative, so it all counts toward your goal. Keep in mind that **it is the regularity, not the intensity, of activity that offers the most protective benefit for your heart.** The more you exercise, the more you improve your personal fitness. If once in a while the regular rhythm of your exercise routine gets altered because you get too busy, go on vacation, or are otherwise interrupted, that's okay. Just be sure to get back on track as soon as you can so *in*activity doesn't become a new habit.

In addition to some type of aerobic activity, another important part of your workout after 50 is strength training (also called resistance training or weight training), which pits your muscles against a force of resistance, such as gravity, weights, or exercise bands. Strength training increases muscle mass, tones and defines individual muscles, increases metabolism, and helps keep weight down as well as improving the stamina and strength of your heart, and thus its pumping ability. Because most women lose 1 percent of muscle mass for every year after menopause, this type of exercise is critical at this stage of life. Another benefit for women in their 50s and older is increased bone density.

Although strength training is a key component of a complete exercise program, it is a complement to—not a replacement for—aerobic exercise. An average healthy but inactive woman in her 50s, should begin strength training with an exercise that involves the major muscle groups of the upper and lower body and do eight to twelve repetitions two days a week. (If you are frail or have heart disease, you can decrease the level of resistance and increase the number of repetitions.)

Need another reason to incorporate physical activity into your life? How about the fact that a regular exercise routine makes you feel good. Chemicals such as endorphins and serotonin are released from the brain into the bloodstream during exercise, resulting in a pain-killing and mood-enhancing effect. When you're exercising, you're doing something beneficial for both your heart *and* your mind . . . and what woman doesn't want to be fit and feel fabulous? Your 50s are the perfect time to commit—or recommit—to building a strong fitness foundation for the decades ahead because it's never too late to improve your heart health.

managing your weight

As your 50-something body starts to sag in new places, you may be thinking you want to lose weight to recapture the body you had at 30. Because of hormonal changes that usually occur in the 50s, it is essential for you to learn how best to manage your weight, but not just for how you look. The key to healthy weight management—especially as you age—is finding the right balance of eating well and exercising regularly.

Fighting Fat in Your 50s

Encroaching weight gain is harder to conquer as you age, so the temptation in your 50s may be to give in and give up. Instead, you need to fight back! Being overweight, *especially* as you get older, is not just a cosmetic problem. **Carrying around extra pounds**—even 10 or 20—**is hard work for your body.** It may not sound like a lot of extra weight, but think about what you have lifted or carried in that weight range, such as an infant, a sack of potatoes, a bag of gardening mulch, or a small dog or large cat. Now think about carrying that around with you all the time. That extra weight puts added strain on all your systems, especially your cardiovascular network. **Extra weight causes your heart to beat harder to pump blood throughout your body, resulting in increased blood pressure.** Statistically, even a moderate amount of excess weight increases the risk of death, particularly among women between 30 and 64 years of age.

It's also a fact that **as you age your percentage of body fat compared to muscle gradually increases.** (This is even truer for women than for men.) As your body composition makes this shift, your metabolism slows down, so you need fewer calories to maintain normal metabolic processes. So, if you've noticed the pounds creeping up on you lately, you're not alone. The average woman gains about 12 pounds in the first four years after she goes through menopause. If you weigh 140 pounds at 50 and gain just 3 pounds a year, by the time you're 65 you'll weigh 185 pounds!

At menopause, you stop producing the female hormone estrogen. The loss of estrogen triggers many changes, including the redistribution of body fat. You may have noticed more fat around your abdomen, whether you've gained extra weight or not. You may hate the bump of fat that protrudes over the top of your jeans, but it's actually the fat *under* the belly's surface that should concern you because that's what poses a real health risk. Visceral fat, the fat that surrounds the abdominal organs, has been linked to cardiovascular disease, diabetes, and other health problems. This fat can create an inflammatory process within the lining of your arteries, putting you at risk for increased atherosclerosis, which then in turn puts you at a higher risk for heart attack or stroke. This is why

keeping your waistline measurement less than 35 inches is so important.

As much as you may want to, however, you can't totally blame the loss of estrogen for the changes in your body composition. Aging and lifestyle are two of the major culprits. Studies have shown that many women tend to be less active as they get older. You might be inclined to let go a little after 50, thinking you can live with those first 10 menopausal pounds. Unfortunately, **your metabolism will continue to slow,** and those 10 pounds may be only the first gain. The extra pounds can add up to hit 20 and then 30—unless you do something to change your pattern of weight gain.

Your 50s can be a turning point when you lay a solid foundation for confronting the health issues of your later years. Your 30s and 40s are behind you, and the genes you inherited have played their part in the background. Now and on through your 60s, however, the major risk factors for heart disease are most likely to show themselves. It's a cumulative process—your blood pressure and your cholesterol and triglyceride levels rise. In fact, from 55 on, the percentage of women with high blood pressure continues to increase. You are more prone to develop diabetes, and you are less inclined to exercise. All the while, if you continue to gain weight, you put your heart under even more stress. It's a perfect storm of interrelated conditions that can lead to a future of ongoing heart trouble and other serious health consequences.

With so much on the line, the 50s is the time to get serious if you want to battle the bulge. You can't rely on a crash diet to lose 10 pounds the way you might have in your 20s. You need to rethink your weight-control strategies to counteract the change in metabolism you're facing, especially if your eating habits have not been exemplary in the past and you have not incorporated a regular routine of physical activity into your lifestyle.

Assess Your Eating Habits

As your body changes, you'll need to **balance your daily food intake with the energy your body is burning.** It's a simple equation: calories in = calories out. To do this, first assess your current eating habits. Are the foods you choose providing you with the nutritional value you need? Do you rely on too many convenience foods that are high in saturated fat, cholesterol, and sodium?

To assess your calorie intake, write down everything you eat and drink for a week, and record the time you spend on physical activity. At the end of the week, calculate your average daily calorie count. Refer to the box in Appendix C to determine the number of calories you can eat each day to maintain your current weight. Compare that number with your actual daily calorie average. If your actual daily calorie intake is more than what you need to maintain your weight, you will gradually gain weight. If you need to lose weight, you will need to find ways to subtract calories from your daily average.

If your usual eating habits are adding extra pounds, make a plan that will allow you to decrease your intake of calories and increase your activity level to provide you with a healthy balance.

Here are some helpful weight-management techniques:

- **Eat smaller amounts** of high-calorie, low-nutrient foods.

- **Plan wisely for cravings.** If you need to feed your chocolate craving, try a square of dark chocolate rather than a candy bar. You can save yourself a couple hundred calories, if not more.

- When you eat out, plan to **share your meal or take half your food home.** Most restaurants give you much more food than the recommended serving size.

- **Learn to eyeball your food for healthy portion control.** For example, a serving of poultry or meat should be about the size of a computer mouse or deck of cards.

- **Make simple lower-calorie substitutions for the foods you eat regularly.** Perhaps you'll choose fat-free, sugar-free yogurt instead of low-fat regular yogurt and save yourself about 90 calories. Try a cinnamon-raisin English muffin instead of a cinnamon roll and deduct about 300 calories.

- **Choose a variety of types and colors of vegetables and fruits** to replace higher-calorie foods.

- **Choose heart-healthy sources of unsaturated fat** such as canola and olive oils, nuts, and avocado, but use them sparingly since they are high in calories.

- **Think before you eat,** especially if the food doesn't offer your body much of a healthy payoff. Ask yourself if you really want to spend your calorie allotment on that treat. If the answer is yes, enjoy it without guilt, but cut back on something else later to balance the indulgence.

- **Stop using food as a source of comfort.** When you feel emotional eating kicking into high gear, redirect those emotional energies toward something else. Try meditating, taking a walk, soaking in a bath, reading a novel, or just sitting outside in the sunshine for a short time, which is a great way to get vitamin D.

- **Plan for several small servings of nutritious snacks,** such as a small handful of nuts, fresh or dried fruit, and fat-free cheese, during the day. Such "grazing" can act both to stave off hunger and to keep your metabolism from hitting highs and lows.

- **Do not starve yourself.** Very low-calorie diets may actually *slow* your metabolism even more.

- **Make exercise a priority** and schedule at least 30 minutes of physical activity into your day (60 minutes if you are trying to lose weight). Block time on your calendar just as you would do for a meeting or doctor's appointment.

To manage your weight most effectively, you need to **make every calorie—and every step—count.** If you can prevent middle-age spread and lose any excess weight you have already gained, you can make a big difference in how well you feel and in the health of your heart for years to come.

managing your health care

For most women over 50, along with the outward signs of aging comes the potential diagnosis of some kind of chronic health issue, such as high blood pressure or high cholesterol and triglycerides. The realization that now, more than ever before, you are vulnerable to heart disease may trigger emotions such as denial, anger, sadness, or depression. Although those emotions are normal, it's important to tackle the health realities head on and **feel empowered to take charge of your heart health.**

Recruit a Team of Healthcare Providers

Since the need for more therapeutic health care increases with age, it becomes essential to **establish a strong partnership with healthcare professionals you can trust.** If you haven't established a network of trusted healthcare providers by your 50s, now is the time to make it a priority. Don't wait until you have serious problems to find doctors with whom you feel a rapport and in whom you have confidence. If you are unsure where to start, ask friends or family for recommendations, do research on reliable websites, or contact local hospitals or your insurance company for references.

When building your core team of healthcare professionals, look for doctors with whom you can communicate easily. (For information on how to talk to your doctor, see Appendix B.) Do they ask questions to help assess your health? Do they listen well? Do they explain things clearly? Do they encourage you to ask questions? Ideally, your doctor will give you clear and precise explanations of tests and procedures, a full discussion of risk factors and potential treatments, and the assurance of a sympathetic but realistic ear. On your side, you should provide enough specific information about your symptoms and lifestyle habits to allow for an accurate diagnosis. **Be prepared to be an active partner with your healthcare professional.** If your doctor makes you feel rushed or doesn't communicate clearly, switch to another doctor now.

In your 50s, it's important that you have regular checkups, screenings, and tests to monitor existing risk factors and detect any that may be developing. (For more information on health screening and diagnostic testing, see Chapter 9.)

Managing Risk Factors in Your 50s

No one can predict a future heart attack or a rise in blood pressure, but **the more risk factors you have, the more likely you are to develop some kind of heart-health problem.** In addition to the risks posed by physical inactivity and obesity/overweight, the risk factors you most likely will need to manage in your 50s include high blood pressure, high LDL cholesterol, high triglycerides, and diabetes. (For more information on these and other risk factors, see Chapter 2.)

HIGH BLOOD PRESSURE

Now that you are in your 50s, you may notice your blood pressure creeping up. Women are more likely to develop high blood pressure after menopause, and almost 30 percent of women have high blood pressure by the time they reach 55. (More men than women have high blood pressure until the age of 45. From ages 45 to 54, the percentages are similar. However, after 54 years, a much higher percentage of women than men have high blood pressure.) Although measures to control blood pressure are available, high blood pressure seems to be an increasing problem in women. **Have your blood pressure checked every time you go to see one of your healthcare providers**—even if you are just there for a sore throat. Be sure to ask what your numbers are, know what they should be, and watch them closely. High blood pressure is often referred to as the "silent killer" because people who have it show no obvious symptoms. A blood pressure check is the only way to determine whether your blood pressure is normal. Regular physical activity and a low-sodium diet that emphasizes vegetables and fruits, whole grains, and fat-free and low-fat dairy products can help you lower your blood pressure. If these steps don't work, however, your doctor may prescribe medication.

HIGH LDL CHOLESTEROL AND HIGH TRIGLYCERIDES

High levels of LDL cholesterol in your bloodstream increase your risk for heart disease by contributing to the accumulation of plaque along vessel walls. The older you are, the more time plaque has had to collect, narrow and damage your arteries, and slow the flow of blood, which puts more stress on your heart. Your target LDL level will depend on what other risk factors you may have.

High triglyceride levels may contribute to hardening of the arteries or thickening of the artery walls (atherosclerosis), which also increase the risk of heart attack and heart disease. **Hormonal changes resulting from menopause can affect your cholesterol and triglyceride levels.** Be sure to have periodic blood tests to determine your total cholesterol, LDL cholesterol, HDL cholesterol, and triglyceride levels. If diet and exercise are not enough to lower high lipid levels, your healthcare professional may prescribe medication.

DIABETES

Type 2 diabetes usually develops in women after age 45. Because of the loss of certain hormones, postmenopausal women are at higher risk for developing diabetes. There are, however, things you can do to delay or even prevent diabetes, especially if you take action sooner rather than later. **Women with diabetes are two to four times as likely to have heart disease as women without diabetes, and their heart attacks are more often fatal.** Because of cultural influences on diet and other lifestyle factors, African American, Latin American, and Native American women have an even higher risk. Be sure to get a fasting blood glucose screening to determine your risk level. The triad of healthy diet, weight control, and physical activity that will protect you from heart disease will also protect you from developing diabetes.

METABOLIC SYNDROME

A combination of risk factors, metabolic syndrome greatly increases your risk of heart disease. If you have three or more of the risk factors listed below, you are considered to have metabolic syndrome.

- Waist measurement equal to or greater than 35 inches

- Triglyceride level of 150 mg/dL or higher

- HDL cholesterol less than 50 mg/dL

- Systolic blood pressure of 130 mmHg or higher

- Diastolic blood pressure of 85 mmHg or higher

- Fasting glucose reading of 100 mg/dL or higher

. . .

The inevitable reality is that everyone ages, and with aging comes the increased likelihood of having several risk factors for heart disease and a greater need for good health care. You look to your doctors to give you dependable information, discuss the available treatment options with you, and use their professional expertise to advise you on how best to manage your heart health. As an equal partner and active participant, you are responsible for sharing information, keeping records of your medical history, and laying the groundwork for your future medical care.

checklist for achieving heart health in your 50s

✓ **Make your heart health a top priority.**

✓ **Learn to make every calorie count** for good nutrition. Find ways to add vegetables, fruits, and whole grains to your diet.

✓ **Develop a lifestyle plan** that incorporates healthy eating habits and regular exercise into your daily routine.

✓ **Follow the plan** and modify it if necessary.

✓ **Understand how menopause is affecting your body and your heart health.**

✓ **Keep your weight under control** by cutting back on calories and being physically active.

✓ **Maintain a network of trusted healthcare professionals.**

✓ **Get regular health checkups and know your numbers.**

✓ **Be aware of your risk factors and take steps to manage them**—especially smoking, elevated blood pressure, diabetes, unhealthy cholesterol levels, and overweight and obesity.

✓ **Take medications as prescribed** by your healthcare professionals.

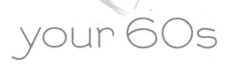

CHAPTER 7

your 60s

. . .

My husband and I recently retired and soon afterwards talked about how we were going to spend our days. We agreed that we needed to keep active—especially since we were "seniors" now. We both have high cholesterol, so we knew it was important for us to exercise to help keep it under control. We joined the community recreation center and go there three to four times a week. I take a senior swim class and a yoga class and also work out with some of the weights. Sometimes I don't have as much energy as I wish I had, but I go anyway. I feel better after exercising and enjoy the interaction with people that I used to get at my job. Plus, I know that I am doing something to protect my heart. —KATHY, 64

. . .

You're going to make choices in your 60s that reinvent your life.

Committing to live a healthy lifestyle can still have a positive impact on your overall well-being and quality of life.

Statistics show that the majority of heart attacks in women occur in the ten years after menopause. **Your risk of heart attack is now equal to that of a man.** Do everything you can to minimize the threat to your heart and maximize your ability to enjoy the years ahead.

Be realistic and optimistic about your health:

- **Eat a balanced diet.** Your tastes and living situation may be changing, but it's still important to include all the food groups, especially vegetables, fruits, and whole grains, for a nutritious diet.

- **Find a type of physical activity you can enjoy and participate in it regularly.** Exercise will help keep your heart muscle, as well as the other muscles and bones in your body, strong.

- If you've been diagnosed with one or more risk factors, **follow your doctor's recommendations for lifestyle changes and take prescribed medications as directed.**

- **Know the warning signs of heart attack and stroke.** Women's signs tend to be less dramatic and harder to diagnose than men's. Listen to your body and seek help at the first sign that something is wrong.

Even if you have developed risk factors for heart disease, think of them as a wake-up call to control the things you can and give yourself the gift of increased vitality.

american heart association
complete guide to women's heart health

introduction

This decade is often a time of renewed choices and reflection. You may choose to continue to work, start a new career, or retire and focus more time and energy on friends, grandchildren, hobbies, and travel. You may choose to move to a different city, downsize, or split your time between two locations. You also may have reflected on what's important, what makes you happy, and what it means to you to be getting older.

By your 60s, your body has been through some natural physical changes that come along with aging. You may be experiencing some new physical limitations. Even if you are starting to feel that age is creeping up on you, don't be discouraged from striving for continued vitality in your life rather than settling for less.

If you are a 60-year-old woman, statistics show that, on average, you can look forward to living about another 20 years or more. You want to make the most of those years, so don't allow a few new wrinkles and an additional ache here or there to keep you from taking care of your health and enjoying a satisfying lifestyle. Of course, you can't stop the physical changes of aging, but you can work around them to sustain your vitality, especially through healthy choices. Thanks to recent research on women's health, you have access to new ways of managing conditions that were considered untreatable only a decade ago.

The 60s are a pivotal decade for a woman's heart health because she is now just as much at risk for a heart attack as a man. Yet because so many of the symptoms of heart disease in women are "silent" or vague, **many women in their 60s already have some form of heart disease without even knowing it.** That's because when women have heart disease, they often don't experience the typical chest pain—caused by angina, or inadequate blood flow to the heart muscle—that men do. Instead, women may feel shortness of breath, dizziness, nausea, or discomfort in one or both arms, chest, or back. These symptoms may come with everyday activities that increase heart rate, such as vacuuming or climbing stairs. If the symptoms go away with rest, they may indicate an underlying condition that reduces blood flow, such as atherosclerosis or congestive heart failure. If they don't go away in a few minutes or if they occur during sleep, these symptoms may signal a heart attack. (For more information on warning signs, see Appendix E.)

Invest in Your Health

Regardless of your current heart-health status, **the more risk factors you can keep under control, the less likely you are to have a future heart attack.** Start by working with your doctor to identify or confirm your existing risks and set up a plan to manage them—and thereby lessen their impact on your health. Second, assess your lifestyle to identify unhealthy behaviors, such as smoking and eating a poor diet, and replace them with healthy ones. The future payoffs of investing in better health should motivate you to take action—*before* you experience the scare of a cardiovascular event.

To get started, make a commitment to care for yourself as well as you care for others. Also **remember that heart disease is not just a man's problem.** If you worry about your husband's or brother's risk of heart attack, for example, remember that you are now as much at risk as he is. If you encourage your partner to watch his high cholesterol or blood pressure levels, let that remind you to get yours checked too. If someone in your family has diabetes, get regular glucose screenings to monitor your blood sugar. And if unhealthy lifestyle habits, such as eating poorly and being inactive, have contributed to that person's higher risk, you need to consider whether you share similar habits that put you at risk as well.

As part of your commitment to good health, be sure to communicate openly and honestly with your healthcare provider, especially if you experience a symptom that is out of the ordinary. Many women in their 60s delay getting treatment because they don't want to make a fuss over nothing or they're afraid to find out something's wrong. Don't be one of them. Whatever the reason, if you know you have a tendency to procrastinate, recognize it and fight it. Otherwise, the consequence could be a heart attack or stroke.

Your health is an important investment and should be a top priority. Whether you're 60 or 69, **leading a healthy lifestyle that includes good nutrition, regular physical activity, and weight management is the best way to maintain your vitality and zest for life.** Even if you've hit a few bumps along the way, it's never too late to make effective changes in your lifestyle and in your attitude—changes that will bring you better heart health and a better quality of life.

Your heart-health priorities for your 60s are to:

- **Pay attention to good nutrition.** Include a wide variety of foods. You need nutrients and fiber from all the foods groups, and the best way to get them is to avoid getting in a food rut.

- **Make physical activity a priority.** If regular exercise hasn't been a routine part of your life, make it one now. Get your heart rate up and keep your blood pumping and your heart strong. If you need to modify your activities to match your capabilities, experiment to find something you enjoy, then stick with it.

- **Maintain a healthy weight.** Keep your calorie needs in balance with your calorie intake. Guard against the temptation to eat for comfort and to become less active, a double whammy for weight gain in the 60s.

- **Manage your risks.** Know the risk factors you are facing and follow the recommendations of your healthcare team to keep them
  under control. Lifestyle changes will make a big difference in
  reducing your risk of heart attack and keeping your medications
  to a minimum.

- **Actively partner with your doctor.** Jointly monitor your heart
  health and maintain good communication. Be proactive about
  scheduling checkups, and communicate to your healthcare team
  any new symptoms or concerns that might signify a developing
  risk factor. Follow your doctor's recommendations for diet and
  exercise, and take medications as prescribed.

- **Learn the signs of heart attack and share them with your
  friends.** The movie-version heart attack is not accurate for many
  women, and the stereotype does women a disservice because it
  keeps them from getting early diagnosis and treatment.

eating for a healthy heart

If you are already eating a generally healthy diet, you are off to a great
start, especially if the calories you consume are in balance with the calories you burn and you are getting all the nutrients your body needs. If,
however, your eating habits have gone off track (or never were on track),
it's time to put a premium on eating right for the sake of your heart.

Putting Nutrition First

Eating well is a vital part of good health. Poor eating habits result in
poor nutrition, increasing the risk for conditions such as heart disease and
osteoporosis. On the flip side, good nutrition can lessen the effects of conditions such as high blood pressure, diabetes, osteoporosis, and even existing heart disease. If your overall eating pattern could use an overhaul, ask
yourself what is motivating your food choices. Are you eating differently
because you no longer need to cook for a family and it just doesn't seem
worth the trouble for one or two people? Are you so tired at the end of

the day that you'd rather eat out than spend time in the kitchen? Have you started relying more on convenience foods instead of buying fresh produce, fish, and meats? Is eating well simply not a top priority? If you answered "yes" to any of these questions, you may need to make some important changes in your eating pattern, because what you eat does make a difference in your 60s. **It's never too late to benefit from good nutrition,** and it's time to turn poor eating habits into healthier ones.

Extensive research has shown that **making the right dietary changes—such as adding vegetables, fruits, and whole grains— can have a profound effect on heart disease risk.** Well-known and respected therapeutic eating plans, such as the DASH (Dietary Approaches to Stop Hypertension) diet, focus on increasing consumption of vegetables and fruits, whole grains, and fat-free and low-fat dairy products while reducing saturated and trans fats and dietary cholesterol. Your healthcare professional may recommend a particular eating plan if you have high blood pressure, high cholesterol, or other risk factors for heart disease. Most plans are very similar to the following dietary recommendations of the American Heart Association, which were developed by expert consensus to provide essential nutrients while helping reduce risk. For the most complete range of nutrients, include a variety of choices from all these food groups in your diet.

A healthy diet includes:

- **A variety of vegetables and fruits.** To get the benefit of the many nutrients provided by vegetables and fruits, including vitamins and minerals, it's important to eat a wide assortment, and especially to include the deeply colored ones. Many vegetables and fruits contain nutrients that can't be replaced by a multivitamin supplement or that provide added benefits in combination with certain other nutrients in foods. Vegetables and fruits also are an excellent source of fiber. Aim to eat at least four or five servings of both vegetables and fruits every day if your calorie needs are 2,000 per day. If you require more or less than 2,000 calories, adjust the number of servings accordingly.

- **Whole-grain and high-fiber foods.** Whole grains are another source of important nutrients, including fiber. Eating whole grains helps keep harmful LDL cholesterol levels down and may lower your risk for coronary heart disease and diabetes. Although whole grains are an essential part of a balanced diet at any age, researchers have found that they may be even more beneficial as you age. In fact, according to one study, older adults who consumed more whole grains significantly lowered their risk of having metabolic syndrome, a combination of factors that increases risk for cardiovascular disease (and is described near the end of this chapter). Choose from whole-wheat breads, whole-grain pastas, brown rice, and whole-grain cereals. When shopping, look for labels that list whole grain as the first ingredient. Try to eat about 21 grams of fiber a day if you are eating a 2,000-calorie diet. Begin the day with a breakfast that includes a half cup of 100 percent bran cereal (9 grams of fiber) and one cup of strawberries (3 grams), for example. Then throughout the day look for ways to incorporate more fiber by adding high-fiber foods such as kidney beans, chickpeas, green peas, or cooked mixed vegetables.

- **Fat-free and low-fat dairy products.** Fat-free and low-fat milk, cheeses, yogurt, and other dairy foods are good sources of calcium. Both to help your heart and, by slowing the rate at which osteoporosis develops, to protect your bones, make sure you get enough of this important nutrient. In your 60s, you should aim for three servings of dairy foods a day to reach a total of about 1,200 mg of calcium. For example, you could have a cup of fat-free yogurt (about 450 mg), a 3-ounce slice of fat-free cheese (about 350 mg), 3 ounces of canned pink salmon (about 120 mg), and an 8-ounce glass of fat-free milk (about 300 mg). (If you have trouble digesting milk or do not like the taste of it, try lactose-free or reduced-lactose milk products; low-fat soy-based beverages, yogurts, ice creams, and cheeses; and tofu or fortified orange juice.) Because vitamin D helps your body use calcium, it is generally added to milk products. You may want to talk to your healthcare provider about also taking calcium and vitamin D supplements to be sure you are meeting your body's needs. In addition to calcium, dairy products are an excellent source of meatless protein.

- **Fish rich in omega-3 fatty acids.** Omega-3 fatty acids provide several benefits that help keep your heart healthy. They can slow the progression of atherosclerosis and help lower levels of LDL cholesterol and triglycerides. Omega-3 fats also may help prevent blood clots from forming and reduce the risk for problems in heart rhythm. Aim for at least two 3-ounce servings (cooked weight) of fish every week, especially the fatty fish that are rich in omega-3, such as salmon, trout, and tuna. Count the fish as part of your daily protein intake (see the next paragraph). Also, ask your doctor whether taking a fish oil supplement would be beneficial.

- **Lean poultry and meats.** When incorporating poultry and meats into your eating plan, choose skinless white-meat chicken and turkey and lean cuts of meat, including sirloin, eye-of-round, and pork tenderloin, and keep portions to about the size of a deck of cards. For a well-balanced meal, visualize your plate divided into four parts: vegetables in two parts, a whole grain in another, and a serving of meat, poultry, or seafood in the fourth. Aim for no more than 6 ounces of cooked lean poultry or meat (about 8 ounces raw) a day. That may be less than you think; restaurant portions for one entrée may easily exceed that amount. You need only about 50 grams of protein daily, so having 1 cup of fat-free yogurt (9 grams), 3 ounces of cooked chicken breast (about 25 grams), and 3 ounces of cooked pork loin chop (about 24 grams) provides more than enough for one day. If you have high cholesterol, limit your intake of meats and poultry to 5 ounces or less a day.

- **Legumes, nuts, and seeds.** Legumes, such as beans, lentils, chickpeas, and peanuts, are a valuable nutritional source of fiber and vegetable protein and do not contain the saturated fat and cholesterol found in meats and poultry. Try including some vegetarian meals as part of your eating plan to help reduce your blood cholesterol levels. A small handful of nuts or seeds, such as walnuts, almonds, and sunflower seeds, will make a satisfying snack or topping and are rich in unsaturated fats, which can help reduce LDL cholesterol and blood pressure. (Some nuts, such as macadamia and Brazil, are high in saturated fat, so use them sparingly.)

- **Healthy unsaturated oils and fats.** Nutrition experts recognize unsaturated oils as an essential part of a healthy diet. Canola, olive, and soybean oils are high in the beneficial fats, omega-3 and omega-6, that can help keep LDL cholesterol low and reduce triglyceride levels. All fats are high in calories, so be sure the amount you consume fits within your calorie needs.

In addition to knowing what foods to include in your diet, it's important to know what to limit. To help you gauge how certain foods fit into your eating plan, use these guidelines as you make your food choices.

- **Aim to limit sodium to less than 1,500 mg a day.** Middle-aged women, especially African Americans and women with high blood pressure, need less than the 2,300 mg recommended for healthy young adults.

- **Aim to limit cholesterol to less than 300 mg each day.**

- **Aim to limit saturated and trans fats as much as possible.** Try to be sure that your intake of these harmful fats does not reach an unhealthy proportion of your daily calorie intake.

IF YOU USUALLY EAT THIS MANY CALORIES EACH DAY					
	1,200	1,500	1,800	2,000	2,500
Keep **saturated fat** to less than	9 grams	11 grams	13 grams	15 grams	19 grams
Keep **trans fat** to less than	1 gram	1.5 gram	2 grams	2 grams	2.5 grams

If you are now living with risk factors such as high blood pressure, high cholesterol, or diabetes, you may have certain limitations on your diet, including how much sodium, cholesterol, or saturated fat you should consume. At the same time, in your 60s you want to be sure you get enough calcium and other important nutrients. Potassium, for example, is important in regulating blood pressure. Potassium-rich foods include bananas, orange juice, and spinach. Magnesium, found in foods such as green leafy vegetables, nuts, and beans, is another essential mineral that is often lacking in women's diets. Ask your healthcare provider whether you should consider taking supplements, such as fish oil or vitamin D, to complement your diet.

Eating Smart

To suit your age, lifestyle, and health concerns, you'll need to tailor your eating plan to your current needs. To start, ask yourself what kinds of foods you eat on a regular basis. Do they provide you with the best health payoff, or do you eat a lot of junk food or convenience food with little nutritional value? To find out what aspects of your eating routine may need to be modified and which ones are working, you need to evaluate your eating habits.

Start by writing down *everything* you eat and drink for a seven-day period. (See the sample food diary page in Appendix C.) Next to each item, make a note of the meal or time of day and whether you ate because of anything besides hunger, such as stress or depression. At the end of the week, review your food journal for patterns and evaluate your results. Are you eating the recommended amounts of vegetables, fruits, and grains each day? Are you eating too many foods high in saturated and trans fats, cholesterol, and sodium? Are you eating too much to maintain a healthy weight? The answers to these questions will help you decide what triggers unhealthy habits, what foods you need to cut back on, and what foods to eat more often. Remember that **it is the overall pattern of your choices that counts the most.** Even if you're already careful to eat well, you probably can do some fine-tuning. If your food journal yielded eye-opening results, however, now is the time to make a fresh start and switch to a more healthy way of eating.

Here are some ideas to help you eat well for a healthy heart in your 60s:

- When cooking your favorite entrées, **make more than you need for one meal.** Freeze individual portions of the extra amount to have healthy, easy meals on hand for days when you do not have the time or energy to cook.

- **Set up a dinner swap with two friends.** Prepare an entrée that freezes well and yields six portions. Wrap the portions individually, then date and freeze them. Keep two and exchange the other four with your friends. Having individual portions gives you the flexibility to serve one or two people.

- **Buy fruits and vegetables any way you prefer**—fresh, frozen, or canned. Frozen and canned fruits and vegetables are packed just after being harvested, at the height of their nutritional value. Make sure canned fruit is packed in water or juice rather than syrup; frozen and canned vegetables should have no or very little sodium added.

- If fresh berries tend to spoil before you can eat all in the package, **freeze part to use in smoothies or chilled fruit soup.**

- **If you use convenience foods** with saturated or trans fats or added sodium, **look for the ones that offer the most nutritional value with the fewest health pitfalls.** For instance, seasoned bread crumbs are handy for breading skinless chicken breasts for baking, but they are very high in sodium. Instead, buy plain bread crumbs, panko, or matzo meal and add dried herbs. Nutrition should always trump convenience.

- **Keep nutrient-rich snacks,** such as low-sodium whole-wheat crackers, peanut butter, fat-free or low-fat cheese, and low-sodium soup, **readily available** at work and at home.

- **Learn some healthy, no-recipe tricks for getting an easy nutrition boost in your food.** Just a few examples are to add a handful of bagged prewashed spinach to salads, soups, stews, pastas, and omelets—even to hamburgers and meat loaf—to provide a flavor and nutrition punch. Or try no-salt-added canned chickpeas in fat-free, low-sodium beef broth for a high-protein snack or light meal when your energy is low.

- **Limit high-fat and high-sugar snacks,** including cake, candy, chips, and soda.

- **Drink plenty of water or water-based fluids** even if you don't feel thirsty. Keep in mind that the older you are, the less well your body registers thirst. If you don't like water, try caffeine-free tea and coffee, soup, and fat-free or low-fat milk; all count as water-based fluids.

- If you're watching your sodium intake, **replace the salt with fresh or dried herbs and spices** to flavor foods. Look in the grocery store for a variety of salt-free seasonings, too. Be sure to give your palate some time to adjust to the lack of salt flavor—it can take up to three months. Salt can mask the taste of food, so once it's been consistently reduced, you'll gradually notice the full flavors of food coming through.

- **Save money by shopping with a friend or family member and sharing perishable items that you can buy in bulk,** such as a large bunch of broccoli, bag of spinach, or head of cabbage.

Nutrition experts agree that the more thoughtfully you choose the foods you eat, the more you can control the risk factors that lead to heart disease and the less likely you'll be to face a life-threatening heart attack. No matter what your age or where you are on the health spectrum, eating wisely is still one of the best choices you can make.

maintaining an active lifestyle

By your 60s, you've maneuvered through menopause, your body shape most likely has shifted some, and perhaps you're experiencing some joint stiffness and a few new aches and pains. You may just feel tired overall. If you're overweight or have coronary heart disease, you may feel winded when you exert yourself. All these factors leave you vulnerable to settling into very sedentary habits, but resist the temptation! **There may not actually be a fountain of youth, but research shows that staying**

physically active can be like finding one. Thus, it's important to find an activity that gets you moving and keeps you moving. Just a 10-minute walk can be the catalyst that energizes you and motivates you to step in the right direction for a lifestyle change.

How Your Heart Is Changing

Your body's capacity for strenuous exercise decreases by about 50 percent between your 20s and 80s. About half this decline is due to the physical changes that take place in your heart itself. Your heart doesn't just weaken with age; it actually adjusts over time in response to the stress of pumping harder as your arteries gradually stiffen and become less elastic. For example, the walls of the left ventricle become thicker so the stress on that muscle is spread over a larger area. The first noticeable results are a lower maximum heart rate and lower cardiac output, which is the amount of blood pumped. Because your heart is a flexible muscle, it will change in shape and size to accommodate your body's demands for oxygen-rich blood. While you are sitting, your heart is "at rest" and can more or less match the cardiac output of a younger heart. However, during exercise or stress, when your body requires a greater output of blood and energy, your heart compensates by growing larger so it can pump a larger volume of blood. Over time, the higher pressure required to move blood effectively gradually forces the heart to work harder, and ventricle walls will continue to thicken. As a result, less oxygenated blood can be pumped through your body, and you may begin to feel short of breath when you exert yourself, by climbing stairs, for example. Like many other aspects of aging, these changes in the heart's capacity occur at a very individual rate.

Why Exercise Is So Important to Your Health

By your 60s, your metabolism has slowed down, and menopause may have left you with a thickening middle section—both reasons to make participating in regular physical activity an important health goal. Weight control is only part of the picture, though. Regular exercise of an intensity that matches your fitness level has health benefits on many fronts. It will boost your energy level and self-esteem as well as improve your overall fitness and strength. Both weight-bearing exercise and strength training will counteract the loss of muscle tone and bone mass you may have already experienced. From 30 to 60 years of age, muscle mass gradually decreases, and the rate of loss accelerates dramatically after age 60. In fact, by age 60, the average woman loses between 10 and 15 percent of her peak muscle mass. **Aerobic exercise will strengthen your heart and lungs and help reduce your risk of heart attack and stroke.**

New study results indicate that **physical activity could help slow the progression of existing heart disease.** Exercise stimulates cells to produce nitric oxide, a natural chemical that helps arteries dilate, thereby promoting the healing of arterial damage caused by the buildup of plaque. Continuing research will add to the understanding of how exercise can help fight heart disease.

Regular physical activity will:

- help you maintain a healthy weight

- reduce arterial stiffening

- lower blood pressure

- reduce harmful LDL cholesterol and increase helpful HDL cholesterol

- reduce the risk of diabetes

- slow the rate of bone loss that occurs after menopause

- strengthen heart muscle and increase cardiovascular capacity

- increase endurance and flexibility

- improve circulation and increase the delivery of oxygen and nutrients to your body's cells

- boost confidence and elevate mood

If you are sedentary and unsure of how much activity is safe for you, or have a condition that affects your ability to exercise, talk with your doctor to work out a reasonable plan that matches your individual capabilities and circumstances before you start an exercise program. Healthy older adults who are fit and have no limiting chronic conditions generally do not need to consult a healthcare provider before becoming physically active.

How Much and What Kind of Exercise?

Aerobic exercise uses large muscle groups to increase your heart rate. The **recommended goal for cardiovascular fitness is at least 150 minutes** (2 hours and 30 minutes) **of moderate-intensity aerobic physical activity a week or 75 minutes** (1 hour and 15 minutes) **of vigorous-intensity activity,** or an equivalent combination of moderate and vigorous activities according to your schedule and preferences. Examples of moderate-intensity aerobic activities include walking briskly (you can speak a few words, but it's difficult to carry on a long conversation), water aerobics, energetic housework or gardening, and ballroom dancing. Examples of vigorous activities are jogging, heavy gardening (digging or hoeing), singles tennis, and swimming laps. Aerobic activity should be performed in episodes of at least 10 minutes, and preferably it should be spread out through the week. Warming up before moderate- or vigorous-intensity aerobic activity by stretching allows for a gradual increase in heart rate and breathing. When done properly, stretching before and after exercise also can increase your flexibility.

If you're not sure how active you are now, try wearing a pedometer for a week and record the number of steps you take each day. If your average is between 5,000 and 7,000 steps a day, you are moderately active. To be considered very active, you need to log at least 10,000 steps a day. From 2,000 to 4,000 steps is considered sedentary.

Here are some sample suggestions for one week:

- Walk at a brisk pace for 35 minutes a day on two days and swim for 20 minutes on two other days.

- Work out with a 30-minute DVD of moderate cardiovascular difficulty five times a week.

- Swim vigorously or jog for 20 minutes on four days.

- Walk around your office building or in the mall fast enough to raise your heart rate; add more walks or other aerobic activity to meet the 30-minute recommendation.

For the greatest health benefit, you'll want to combine aerobic conditioning with some kind of strength training and weight-bearing exercise. Strength training (also called resistance training), which pits your muscles against a force of resistance such as gravity, weights, or exercise bands, helps maintain your muscle mass and strengthen your bones. Examples include lifting weights (start slowly, with 2- or 3-pound weights) and doing household or garden tasks that require lifting or digging. If you have access to the facilities at a gym, have a trainer explain which machines and equipment options are best for you. Easy and inexpensive ways to get a workout at home include using filled water bottles as weights and working with inflatable balance balls and resistance bands. Try to add strength training to your workout at least twice a week.

Weight-bearing activities also require your bones and muscles to work against gravity. They include any activities in which your feet and legs are bearing your total body weight, such as walking, jogging, and playing tennis, and help counteract the loss of bone mass that can occur after menopause. Your bones continue to "remodel" themselves throughout your life, maintaining a balance between loss of bone mass and the rebuilding process. If the rate of bone loss outstrips the rebuilding, osteoporosis results. That's a serious concern because about 50 percent of women older than 50 will have one osteoporosis-related fracture during their lifetime.

In addition to helping rebuild bone and muscle, resistance and weight-bearing exercises help increase your stamina; sturdier bones and muscles and more stamina, in turn, enable you to do many of the everyday things you need to do, such as carrying heavy groceries or strenuous vacuuming. Both types of exercise also develop stronger ligaments and tendons, which tend to weaken with age.

For a well-rounded routine that will also improve balance and help prevent falls as you get older, add activities that require use of your core muscles (abdominals and back) and legs. Yoga, dancing, and tai chi are some examples, and they also incorporate flexibility and stretching, which increase the length of your muscles and improve your range of motion, into your exercise plan.

Be sure to listen to your body and modify or change any activity as needed so that you don't develop a chronic injury. For example, if your knees are starting to hurt when you jog, try swimming. If tennis is too hard on your wrist now, go dancing. You need to modify your exercise routine to match your capabilities, but don't let the need for change keep you from enjoying a full range of activities. Try something new and see how it feels.

Exploring Different Fitness Options

The biggest predictor of whether you'll stick with an exercise routine is whether you enjoy it. To get moving and keep moving, start with a physical activity or two that give you physical benefits as well as emotional satisfaction and that fit into your personal lifestyle.

Try these suggestions:

- **Take short walks throughout your day.** Try a 10-minute walk around your neighborhood with your dog before breakfast, replace a coffee break at work with an exercise break by walking around the office for 10 to 15 minutes, and walk around the local mall or on the local walking trail with a neighbor after dinner.

- **Join a water aerobics or yoga class,** especially if you need a workout routine that's easier on your joints.

- **Take a dip.** Swimming helps strengthen the muscles, tendons, and ligaments that support your joints, improving stability and flexibility.

- Clean your house or garage, mow your lawn and do some gardening, or wash your car instead of hiring someone to do these tasks. **Attack the chores with enough vigor and purpose to get your heart pumping.**

- **Take ballroom dance classes.** A recent study showed that waltzing with a partner on a regular basis can provide as much heart-health benefit as more conventional exercise options.

- **Schedule several 5-minute exercise breaks** at work or when you travel. Stand up and stretch, practice standing on one foot, and roll your shoulders. Sit down in your chair and do 10 leg lifts with each leg.

> Keep up your exercise routine even when you travel. Pack resistance bands to keep up your strength training and a pair of good walking shoes for some aerobic activity while you are away. Also, be sure to take advantage of hotel workout facilities or the passes to local gyms that they may offer.

- **Walk on a treadmill or cycle on a stationary bike.** Both reduce the chance of a fall on uneven outdoor surfaces and can be used rain or shine.

- **Keep some resistance bands** near the television **and use them to stretch** while you're watching your favorite shows.

- **Find ways to add activity "bonuses" to your day.** For example, use the stairs instead of elevators when you can, and pick up the pace when going up or down. At home, sort loads of laundry into smaller batches so you take more trips on the stairs. When parking your car, choose a spot farther away from your destination.

Just Do It

Does the idea of exercise make you cringe? If you haven't exercised in a while, it may be difficult to get started. However, once you begin moving, you'll gain momentum and exercising will become easier. **Start where you're comfortable. Any exercise is an improvement over none,** and you soon will be stronger and able to do more. When it becomes routine to exercise, you've developed a habit that is part of your lifestyle.

An important part of getting started is being positive. Instead of thinking that exercise will be a chore, think: "I will feel energized after I exercise" or "I will walk farther today than I did three days ago." Set short-term goals, write them down, and reward yourself with nonfood treats for achieving them. On days when you don't feel like exercising, ease your way into it. First, put on your workout clothes. Then tell yourself you'll exercise for just 10 minutes. Once you get moving, however, chances are you will do more than you expect. If you allow yourself to take small steps, the idea of exercising won't seem so overwhelming. Scientific studies tell us that the more successful you feel at meeting your fitness goals, the more motivated you are to exercise. As you begin to see results, enjoy the rewards of your efforts and let them be your personal motivation. (Use the activity diary in Appendix C to record your progress.)

managing your weight

Losing weight and keeping it off can be a challenge at any age, but the older you get, the harder it can become. Through the years, your metabolism gradually slows down, you tend to become more sedentary, and you lose muscle. Less physical activity and muscle loss both mean fewer calories burned, which further increases the tendency to gain weight. If you still eat now the way you did in your 20s, or even your 30s or 40s, you will most likely have gained weight—even if you are still doing the same amount of exercise. The bottom line is that **the older you get, the fewer calories your body burns.** That's why managing your weight is even more important now that you are in your 60s.

Being overweight or obese not only jeopardizes vitality but also is a risk factor for heart disease. Extra weight on your body increases the workload on your heart and contributes significantly to other risk factors for disease, such as high blood pressure, high cholesterol, diabetes, and metabolic syndrome. Studies show that **body weight has a big impact on quality of life for people over 65.** For instance, in a survey of more than 7,000 men and women, researchers found that excess body weight was associated with worse overall health for both men and women. Women in particular found it more difficult to perform daily tasks such as climbing stairs or carrying groceries when overweight, and they were less likely to engage in social activities with family and friends. The heavier the participant, the worse the quality of life. **Maintaining a healthy weight will help lessen or manage the effects of existing risk factors**—perhaps even to the extent that medications can be reduced or discontinued. Achieving a healthier weight also comes with the added bonuses of increased energy and self-confidence.

Focus on High Nutrition, Not Just Low Calories

Effective weight control comes when you can balance the amount of food you eat with the calories you burn through exercise and your body's metabolic processes. It's a simple equation: **calories in = calories out.** To make every calorie work best for you, **choose foods that provide your body with maximum nutrition.** Foods that are high in calories but low in nutrients, such as most cakes, candy, and pastries, for example, may be very appealing but quickly tip the scales toward overweight and obesity and don't contribute much, if anything, toward good nutrition. Healthy weight management is twofold: eating the right amount of wholesome food for your body and exercising regularly to burn the calories you have consumed.

Assess Your Eating Patterns

What are your typical eating patterns now? Do you eat balanced meals and healthy snacks? Perhaps you have drifted into less healthy habits, such as eating a bag of light popcorn for dinner. Although this snack-turned-dinner is low in calories, you are missing an opportunity to feed your body with more nutritious foods. If you have a tendency to soothe your nerves with a nice cup of tea and a slice of chocolate cake, you are using up your calorie reserves in a way that's less than optimal for your overall nutrition.

To assess your calorie intake, write down the calorie count for everything you eat and drink for a week, and keep track of time spent on physical activity. At the end of the week, calculate your average daily calorie count. Refer to the box on page 253 to determine the number of calories you can eat each day to maintain your current weight. Compare that number with your actual daily calorie average. If your actual daily calorie intake is more than what you need to maintain your weight, you will gradually gain weight. If you need to lose weight, you will need to find ways to subtract calories from your daily average.

Your food diary can also help you understand where you are "spending" your calories. Look for patterns such as too much eating of certain foods and choosing foods that are high in calories. Do you have a lot of sweets and snacks in the house for when the grandchildren come to visit or in case company drops by? The "they're for company" foods can sabotage both your waistline and a balanced eating plan. Do you grab snacks on the run because you're overextended at work? Are you eating for comfort or to combat boredom because you're not quite sure what to do after retirement? Do you have a habit of relaxing in the evenings with a bowl of ice cream while you watch your favorite TV shows? Once you see how you go off track, you can plan ways to sidestep overeating and defuse the triggers with lower-calorie substitutions.

Depression, stress, and grief are common causes for comfort eating that can lead to accumulating weight gain. If you are coping with any of these, talk with your healthcare professional so you can find the best strategy to both deal with your emotions and get your weight back under control.

Get Moving

The more extra weight you carry now, the more sedentary you are likely to become later—and the less vitality you may have. Avoiding physical activity can set in motion a dangerous spiral: you burn fewer calories and continue to allow muscle mass to decrease, and, in turn, increased deposits of fat collect around your abdomen and lungs. The fat around your lungs can cause reduced lung function, which then leads to your feeling more tired and out of breath, which makes exercise even more difficult. Staying active is important because exercise not only helps you burn calories and restore muscle but also strengthens your lungs, offering double benefits for your efforts.

Helpful Weight Control Strategies

Here are some tips to help you manage your weight in your 60s:

- **Focus on portion control to keep calories in check.** Learn how to eyeball a healthy portion by comparing it to the size of a familiar object. For example, a healthy serving of cooked fish, meat, or poultry is about the size of a deck of cards.

- Even if you're not hungry, **do not skip meals.** Skipping meals may cause your metabolism to slow down or lead you to eat more high-calorie, high-fat foods at your next meal or for a snack.

- **Choose lower-calorie alternatives for the high-calorie foods** you eat. For example, if jelly doughnuts are a routine breakfast for you, switch to whole-wheat toast with all-fruit strawberry jam instead.

- **Focus on your food when you are eating.** Studies show that eating while watching television or reading induces people to eat more than if they are less distracted. Even listening to music can lead to automatic eating and more calorie intake than you planned.

- **Be mindful of what you drink.** You may be consuming high-calorie liquids without even realizing it. Whole milk, tea or coffee with sugar, and sugary sodas and fruit juices can add up to hundreds of calories a day.

- **Keep a small portion of nuts,** such as almonds or walnuts, or dried fruit in your purse **for a heart-healthy snack** that will satisfy your hunger when you are out and about.

- **When you eat out, ask for a to-go container at the start of the meal.** If you pack up half your food before you start eating, you'll be less likely to go back on your good intentions of taking the rest home. Most restaurant portions are much larger than you need for one meal.

- **Watch out for high-calorie sugary foods.** Be aware that as your taste buds become less sensitive, sweetness is one of the last tastes to fade, and so may find yourself tempted by sweets even more than before.

- **Savor high-quality foods in small amounts** and pass up the lesser-quality treats. Substitute a small square of excellent dark chocolate for a whole piece of store-bought chocolate cake, for example.

- **Find a weight-loss partner or support group,** join a weight-loss program, or make a mutual encouragement pact with a friend to keep to a healthy but low-calorie eating plan. It's easier to stick to your commitment when you're not alone.

- **Keep moving.** Exercise burns calories and will help you keep off the weight you lose. Make a regular date with a friend to meet at a park or the track at a local school to walk and talk, or do some low-impact workouts, such as biking or swimming, that allow you to burn a lot of calories without jarring movements that can cause injury.

As you work toward your weight goals, **be realistic in your expectations. Being energized and healthy is your priority.** Losing weight shouldn't be as much about how you look as how you feel and how you can best fuel your body to function at peak performance. By managing your weight effectively, you will gain more freedom to live your life fully—whether that means keeping up with your grandkids, going salsa dancing, or perhaps both!

managing your health care

Because of advances in medical research, technological innovations, new developments in drug therapies, and improvements in preventive care, women today can expect less chronic illness and more effective treatment options than their parents, meaning they can live longer and maintain better health and vitality in their later years. However, you may be putting up your own roadblocks to heart attack prevention and treatment, and medical science still has a lot to learn about women's heart health.

Therefore, it's more important than ever for you to learn as much as you can about your own health.

Although your cardiovascular system gradually adapts as you age, it is the cumulative effects of genetics and 60-plus years of life habits—the good, the bad, and the ugly—that determine your risk for heart disease and heart attack. The research that has defined these risks for women is relatively new, so your impressions of and knowledge about your heart health may be dangerously out of date. Maybe you pay more attention to others' health than your own, yet your risk of heart attack is just as real. Like many other women, you may wait too long to get help because you think the problems will go away by themselves or you don't want to be embarrassed by bothering your doctor with a false alarm. If you do have a heart attack, you may not recognize the symptoms because you don't realize that the stereotyped scene—a middle-aged, overweight man clutching his chest in pain—doesn't always apply for women, or perhaps you just don't believe that a heart attack can actually happen to you.

For many years, medical research was conducted primarily in men, with the results then applied to women. It's only recently that science has turned to studying women, and ongoing research is greatly expanding the understanding of how **women's hearts are different from men's.** As a result, the diagnosis and treatment options for heart disease in women are being rapidly updated. Doctors now are better informed about women's risk, and they are better attuned to the inherent difficulties in recognizing and diagnosing cardiovascular conditions and heart attack as they occur in women, including the fact that **women's symptoms of heart attack can be vague and therefore more difficult to pinpoint.**

Even when doctors are aware of these difficulties, they may have trouble making a firm diagnosis for a woman because common investigative procedures may not show the whole story. Angiography, for example, is designed to identify large, bumpy blockages found in the major coronary arteries. In many women, however, plaque is found distributed smoothly throughout the network of *smaller* arteries, so angiograms alone do not detect dangerously reduced blood flow in these women. In this circumstance and others, technology can effectively find developing disease only if it's looking in the right place. Sometimes several diagnostic tools are needed, including a comprehensive assessment based on the results of an electrocardiogram, exercise stress test, and perfusion scan. (See Chapter 9.) About 385,000 women age 65 and older, which represents almost 19 of every 1,000 of these women, have coronary attacks every year. **Although the average age of a first heart attack is 70, you should be proactive in your health care now to avoid becoming one of these statistics.**

Keep Your Healthcare Team Working for You

A key component to maintaining better health and prolonging longer vitality is partnering with a strong network of healthcare professionals. Establishing a good relationship with your healthcare team will allow you to manage existing risk factors for heart disease and quickly identify changes that could signal developing threats to your health.

Good medical care requires a collaborative approach between patient and doctor. If you don't feel comfortable with your doctor and his or her staff, switch. Don't rationalize the situation or make excuses, and don't worry about hurting your doctor's feelings. Instead, do find a doctor with whom you can easily communicate, one who earns your confidence and will listen carefully to you. As part of an effective partnership, you should be prepared to share information about your symptoms and other concerns openly and honestly with your doctor. Write down symptoms, questions, and concerns as they occur. Don't be embarrassed or shy about taking your written list with you. While you are right there in the office, write down the answers and

Changes in the normal pacing of your heart rhythm are called arrhythmias. You may feel heartbeats that seem to pound against your chest, fluttering, skipped beats, or very fast or slow beats. Most arrhythmias are not serious, but it is important to know what is causing these changes in your heart rate to rule out underlying disease. Arrhythmias tend to occur more often as you get older and can be affected by caffeine, chocolate, alcohol, smoking, drugs such as decongestants, or stress. Even when an arrhythmia isn't a sign of a dangerous condition, it can be frightening. If you experience an arrhythmia that is new or concerns you, call your doctor so the cause can be identified.

Aspirin Therapy: What Is Recommended?

Aspirin therapy helps prevent heart attack and stroke by thinning the blood and inhibiting the formation of blood clots, so it reduces the likelihood of a blood clot blocking a blood vessel. But aspirin also increases the risk of gastrointestinal upset and bleeding.

Expert review of the data from the Women's Health Initiative (WHI) study revealed that the benefits of aspirin therapy to prevent heart attack and stroke were strongest in women of 65 years of age and older. In these older women who took aspirin, the incidence of cardiovascular events was cut by one-third compared with the women who took a placebo. For healthy women *younger* than 65, however, the same level of benefit was not observed, yet the gastrointestinal risks remained.

That's why **the American Heart Association recommends that women over 65 consider daily aspirin therapy** (75 mg to 325 mg a day) **to help prevent heart attack and stroke, as long as blood pressure is managed and the risk of gastrointestinal bleeding is outweighed by the benefit.** No matter what your age or health concerns, be sure to talk with your healthcare provider about how to balance the benefit and risk in your personal situation before you begin aspirin therapy.

other information the doctor provides so you'll have concrete information to refer to. For more guidance on how to get the most from your healthcare partners, see Appendix B.

Once you find the right team of healthcare providers, be sure to see them for regular checkups. Don't be tempted to put off your visits to your doctor's office until something hurts so much you can't ignore it. Although fear and anxiety can make you hesitate, it's important to fight through those emotions so you can be an active participant in your own health care. Accept that for your checkups to be effective as you get older, you will need some diagnostic tests. As the number of risk factors increases, the number of diagnostic tests increases as well. (To learn which tests are age appropriate and should be included in your screening visits, see Appendix A.) Remember to keep a record of test results, including blood pressure and cholesterol levels, in a health journal or computerized health record.

Managing Risk Factors in Your 60s

By 60, age itself is now a risk factor for heart attack and stroke. Whether you currently have heart disease or not, you and your doctor need to assess all the risk factors you face and develop effective strategies to manage them. If you are like most other women in their 60s, you are dealing with at least one heart disease risk factor that requires treatment, perhaps two or three. (For more information on heart-related diseases, conditions, and treatments, see Chapter 10.)

HIGH BLOOD PRESSURE

Blood pressure typically increases with age because your heart has to work harder to pump blood through arteries that have become increasingly stiff and occluded. In fact, about 74 percent of women have high blood pressure (greater than 140/90 mmHg) by the time they reach 65 years of age. High blood pressure is known as a silent killer because it has no symptoms and thus often goes undetected. If you are taking a medication for high blood pressure, have your blood pressure level checked when that specific drug should take full effect to be sure you keep your levels under control (less than 120/80 mmHg). When you begin a new medication, ask your doctor when you should return for a follow-up visit.

New research shows that in addition to increasing the risk for heart attack, stroke, heart failure, and kidney failure, uncontrolled high blood pressure can increase risk for a decline in cognitive functions such as short-term memory and verbal ability. You can help keep your blood pressure down by eating a balanced diet rich in vegetables and fruits, avoiding excessive alcohol use, and following a routine of regular physical activity.

African American and Hispanic women are even more susceptible to high blood pressure than Caucasian women. If you are African American or Hispanic, be sure to have your blood pressure checked often, even if you are currently taking medication.

HIGH LDL CHOLESTEROL AND TRIGLYCERIDES

The LDL cholesterol circulating in your blood has been building up as plaque on the walls of your arteries throughout your life. This buildup makes it harder for blood to flow freely and increases the chance that plaque may crack or break off. When a blood clot forms at the site, it can block blood flow altogether, causing either a heart attack or a stroke. By age 60, you probably have developed some accumulation of plaque. As you continue to get older, your level of LDL also gradually increases, further contributing to your risk. Untreated high cholesterol also has been linked with low bone density, suggesting an increased risk for both bone fracture and coronary heart disease. (Refer to the information on page 20 for target levels of cholesterol and triglyceride, and be sure that you know your cholesterol numbers.) If your cholesterol level puts you at risk for heart disease, you should focus on changing to a healthier diet, incorporating regular exercise into your lifestyle, and taking cholesterol-lowering medication if prescribed by your doctor.

High levels of triglyceride, another type of blood fat, also increase your risk for heart disease and are associated with high LDL cholesterol, low HDL cholesterol, and obesity. Calories not used immediately are converted into triglycerides, which are then transported to fat cells to be stored. When your triglyceride level is too high, it can increase blood viscosity (or thickness), making it harder for blood to flow freely. High triglycerides significantly increase your risk of heart attack, even if your blood cholesterol levels are normal. The first approach to treatment for high triglycerides is lifestyle change: lose weight if needed, reduce your intake of saturated and trans fats and dietary cholesterol, avoid alcohol, eat a balanced diet, and make regular physical activity part of your routine. If your triglycerides are very high or you have family history that puts you at additional risk, your doctor may recommend more aggressive treatment such as medication as well.

OVERWEIGHT/OBESITY AND PHYSICAL INACTIVITY

Being overweight or obese is considered a major risk factor for coronary heart disease. Both conditions raise blood pressure, blood cholesterol, and triglyceride levels and lower levels of "good" HDL cholesterol. (HDL cholesterol is linked with lower risk of heart disease and stroke, so reducing HDL tends to raise your risk.) In addition, overweight and obesity can lead to diabetes, which in turn makes a heart attack more likely. Even if other risk factors are not present, obesity by itself increases your odds of developing heart disease by putting extra stress on your heart and blood vessel system.

Being physically inactive over time increases both your tendency to gain weight *and* your risk of coronary heart disease. In fact, the disease risk associated with physical inactivity is comparable to that for high blood cholesterol, high blood pressure, or cigarette smoking. You can dramatically change your level of risk, however, by beginning a regular program of exercise. Talk with your healthcare professional to find the right strategy that will work for you to both lose weight and stay active.

DIABETES

Diabetes, another major risk factor for heart disease, tends to develop with increasing age, and the prevalence of physician-diagnosed diabetes for women age 65 and older is 17 percent. The risk is much higher if you are a woman of color, especially African American, Native American, or Hispanic. If you have diabetes, you are at a higher risk for coronary heart disease, stroke, peripheral vascular disease, and kidney damage. Your doctor can diagnose diabetes with a simple blood test. Eating a healthy diet, being more physically active, and losing weight will lessen your risk of diabetes. Research shows that patients who receive counseling and make these lifestyle changes may reduce their risk by as much as 58 percent.

METABOLIC SYNDROME

The term *metabolic syndrome* refers to a cluster of coexisting risk factors. They include abdominal fat, lipid disorders that contribute to atherosclerosis (high triglycerides, high LDL cholesterol, and low HDL cholesterol), high blood pressure, and insulin resistance or diabetes. The diagnostic criteria for women are:

- Waist measurement equal to or greater than 35 inches

- Triglyceride level of 150 mg/dL or higher

- HDL cholesterol less than 50 mg/dL

- Systolic blood pressure of 130 mmHg or higher

- Diastolic blood pressure of 85 mmHg or higher

- Fasting glucose reading of 100 mg/dL or higher

Metabolic syndrome greatly increases your risk for coronary heart disease. Most women who have metabolic syndrome are overweight, but new research shows that losing weight isn't the only way to fight the problem. Exercise can help you as well. In a long-term study of more than 7,000 women divided into five groups by fitness level, researchers found that metabolic syndrome was more than three times as prevalent in the group with the lowest level of cardiovascular fitness than in the group at the next level of fitness. If you have three or more of the qualifying risk factors listed above, discuss your individual situation with your doctor and design a program of physical activity to reduce your risk.

. . .

If you have any of the risk factors described above, your doctor may prescribe a regimen of lifestyle changes. Additionally, if you are given medication to reduce a risk factor such as high blood pressure or cholesterol, be sure to take it as prescribed and don't stop on your own. Although you can't see or feel their symptoms, these conditions pose a real threat to your heart. If you experience side effects or your reaction to your medications changes, contact your doctor. Depending on your situation, you may want to consider adding specialists to your healthcare team. For help creating a healthful eating plan, schedule an appointment with a dietitian. **If you are managing one or more risk factors for heart disease, consider seeing a cardiologist for treatment.**

To manage your health care effectively, continue to work with your team of professionals to assess your risks and how best to manage them. The choices you make today have a significant impact on the vitality of your years ahead. To make your life as robust as you can, commit to healthy eating habits and regular exercise, manage your weight, and visit your doctors for regular checkups. Embrace these healthy lifestyle changes and take on your 60s and later decades with a renewed zest for life.

checklist for achieving heart health in your 60s

✓ **Commit to living a healthy lifestyle** to protect your vitality.

✓ **Pay attention to nutrition,** not just calories or convenience.

✓ **Establish a plan** to eat better and add regular exercise to your lifestyle.

✓ **Follow the plan** and modify it if necessary.

✓ **Keep your calorie intake in balance with your level of activity.**

✓ **Maintain a network of trusted healthcare professionals.**

✓ **Be an active partner in your health care.** Get regular health checkups and know your numbers.

✓ **Manage your risk factors**—especially elevated blood pressure, unhealthy cholesterol levels, diabetes, and overweight and obesity.

✓ **Follow your doctor's recommendations** for managing risk factors or existing heart disease.

✓ **Take medications as prescribed** by your healthcare professionals.

✓ **Know the warning signs of heart attack and stroke.**

CHAPTER 8

your 70s and beyond

. . .

I had a heart attack several years ago, take medications to control my blood pressure, and use a walker to help me get around, but I don't let any of that slow me down. When the weather is nice, I like to walk outside. It takes me 30 minutes to walk from one end of my block to the other, but that's okay because I'm not looking to win any races at my age. I just know that I feel better moving—even if it's slowly—than sitting in the house all day. It gets me out in the sunshine and I get to see some of my neighbors. —DORIS, 78

. . .

It's never too late to benefit from a heart-healthy lifestyle.

Many women stay healthy and active through their 70s and can look forward to many more years of savoring life. The years may bring limitations and everyone ages differently, but you can still make choices that will increase your energy and overall quality of life.

Although **your senior years definitely carry increased risk for heart disease and heart attack,** the medical community has made great strides in diagnosing and treating these conditions, especially in women. Take advantage of these advances by communicating openly with your doctors about changes in your health and actively participating in your own health care.

Maintain your heart-healthy habits or add new ones:

- **Be sure to eat well,** even if you don't feel hungry—good nutrition fuels your body and helps fight illness.

- **Stay physically active,** even if it's a challenge, to maintain your fitness level and mobility.

- **Do not accept** struggling with stairs, having difficulty carrying groceries, or feeling breathless when vacuuming as signs **that you're "just getting old."** They may be symptoms of an undiagnosed heart condition. Be sure to see your doctor.

- **Know the warning signs of heart attack and stroke.** Women's signs tend to be less dramatic and harder to diagnose than men's. Listen to your body and seek help at the first sign that something is wrong.

- **Do something healthy for yourself.** Remember, doing something for your heart health, such as taking short walks and eating healthy meals, is always better than doing nothing.

introduction

Thanks to decades of advanced medical research, better general health care, and an improved food supply, **getting old isn't what it used to be.** Today's 70-something woman is just as likely to be traveling around the globe or working outside the home as she is to be knitting in a rocking chair. The physical process of aging, however, catches up with everyone, and in different ways. Even if you've been relatively healthy and fit throughout most of your life, you are likely learning your limits and setting different priorities in your 70s—and you are probably managing some risk factors for heart disease as well.

As you are learning to cope with the challenges that come with age, your heart is also undergoing physical changes that help it adapt. Much research has been conducted recently on what aging means, and the medical community now knows that many of the disabilities of age once considered inevitable—such as heart disease—are *not*. Instead of accepting a sedentary lifestyle, loss of energy, and declining health as "typical" at your age, you *can* continue making a real difference in areas within your control: lifestyle and attitude. **By choosing to live healthy and stay upbeat, you are protecting your vitality and independence.**

Think of eating well and being physically active as being major components of your healthcare regimen, and consider them as important as going to your doctor and taking medication. Studies show that these **healthy behavior choices may actually do as much—if not more— good than medicine to maintain the quality of your life well past your 80s,** resulting in a long list of mental and physical benefits. Yet it's only recently, because of an increased and growing understanding of the extent to which women are subject to heart disease and heart attacks, that the medical community has focused on educating older women about the importance of adopting a healthy lifestyle and a positive mindset. As life expectancy for women increases, the message is clear: **it's never too late to take care of yourself.**

In a survey of almost 3,500 seniors over age 65, researchers found that the quality of life for most older women is actually very high. Most of the women surveyed lived independently and felt themselves to be in excellent or good health—even after their 85th birthday. The women who were most likely to report being in good physical health were also those who reported *feeling* healthy. The common denominator was that they were committed to living well, despite dealing with typical setbacks associated with aging, such as losses in hearing or vision. The reassuring implication of this study is that although aging brings many changes, you can meet its challenges head on with a healthy outlook that includes eating for good nutrition, committing to be physically active, and embracing a positive attitude.

Understanding How Your Heart Is Changing

Scientists once assumed that the heart shrank or simply wore out with age, but they now know that aging hearts actually adapt over time. The heart's responses to changes occurring within the aging cardiovascular system, which comprises not only the heart but also the large and small blood vessels throughout the body, can also make the heart more vulnerable. With recent advances in diagnostic technology, researchers have been able to see inside the body to better understand how aging affects your cardiovascular system, and specifically your heart.

As the cardiovascular system ages along with the rest of the body, the walls of your arteries gradually become less elastic, and consequently they become stiffer and less responsive. As a result, your arteries cannot relax as quickly after your heart pumps blood, which results in increased blood pressure. Valves in the heart thicken and also relax more slowly. To keep the blood moving effectively, your heart adjusts with structural changes. For example, the muscular wall of the left ventricle thickens to enhance its pumping action and compensate for increased blood pressure, and the left atrium expands to hold more blood. Over time, the higher pressure required to maintain adequate blood flow forces the heart to work harder. Individual factors such as the elasticity of your arteries and the diameter of these vessels, which may have narrowed over the years because of plaque buildup, all contribute to the workload your heart must overcome during each heartbeat.

The process of atherosclerosis, the accumulation of fatty deposits of plaque on the walls of your arteries, has been occurring since your childhood. The extent of the atherosclerosis is largely dependent on your family history and your lifestyle choices related to diet and exercise over time. With the aging process, your blood pressure may rise as well. In fact, **almost 74 percent of women will have high blood pressure by age 65.** The constant force of high blood pressure combined with plaque buildup in your blood vessels increases your risk for heart disease, heart attack, and stroke. If you also have other significant risk factors such as diabetes, high LDL cholesterol and triglycerides, or excess weight, your risk becomes even greater.

It is also important at this time of life to be mindful of other heart-related conditions described in Chapter 10, such as an arrhythmia (an irregular heartbeat), heart failure (progressive symptoms that show the heart is not pumping effectively), or angina (usually experienced as chest pain with exertion, which goes away with rest). You should also **be aware of the warning signs of heart attack and stroke** (see Appendix E).

Disorders that lessen your heart's efficiency to pump blood may not be life threatening by themselves. But because **it can be difficult to diagnose heart disease in women,** it is especially important to pay attention to signs such as increasing tiredness with routine activities, shortness of breath or difficulty catching your breath, the need for extra pillows to raise your head when sleeping, or unusual swelling in your hands and feet.

It is important to know that women's heart attack symptoms vary enormously, and the pain or discomfort that women experience can be confusing and difficult to evaluate. The good news is that most women *do* experience some warning as their heart disease progresses. **Listen to your body and pay attention to signs and symptoms** because seeking early medical attention will help to minimize heart damage.

Making Good Health a Top Priority

No one really knows why some of us age with fewer cardiac problems than others. Certainly genetics plays a role, and so do the lifestyle habits you've established over the years. If you don't smoke and have been eating well and staying active, you've already improved your chances of better health. If you've lived for many years without paying much attention to how your lifestyle affects your health, you can make it a priority to make changes *now*. It's never too late to improve your quality of life so you can continue to enjoy your favorite activities and reduce your risk of having a heart attack.

So, what can you do? To start, you can make sure to **engage in physical activity and eat a heart-healthy diet,** both of which provide positive benefits to your overall well-being, as well as your cardiovascular health. Regular physical activity may help to lessen the risks posed by high blood pressure and reduce the progression of arterial plaque.

The reality is that some women in their senior years feel they face obstacles that interfere with their desire or ability to make lifestyle changes. What struggles make change difficult for you? Living alone, dealing with chronic pain, adjusting to reduced mobility, and other obstacles can make it hard to keep eating well or being active. Although preparing a healthy meal may not seem worth the effort at the moment, especially if getting to the store is a chore and the taste of food isn't as enjoyable as it once was, the long-term reward is indeed worthwhile. (See "Overcoming Barriers to Eating Well" on page 193 for some helpful tips.)

Keep in mind that your body—no matter at what age—still needs a balance of nutrients to stay healthy, energized, and resistant to illness, and too much of the wrong food may increase your risk of disease. You may not want to prepare the elaborate meals you once did, and that's just fine. Eat simply instead. Go easy on yourself and respect your limits, but **don't stop giving your body the nutritious foods it needs.**

You might wonder why you should start an exercise program now or even continue the one you've been on. It's because **exercise will continue to improve your stamina and energy as well as help ward off disease and heart attack.** If you are afraid that you'll hurt yourself or are daunted because you don't know how to begin, talk with your healthcare provider to overcome these roadblocks so you can incorporate some physical activity into your lifestyle—no matter what your current fitness level or health status is.

Although the average woman is living 30 years longer now than 100 years ago, longevity should not be a goal in itself. **Strive instead to age successfully, to combine quantity *and* quality of life.** Take a minute and think about why it's important to you to stay healthy and vital as you age. Is it so you can continue to live on your own, go out with friends, play with your grandchildren? If you invest your energy in a healthier way of life, these are just some of the personal payoffs you can expect.

Your heart-health priorities in your 70s are:

- **Eat well.** To protect your heart and resist infection and disease, be sure you meet your nutritional needs.

- **Stay active.** Be as active and mobile as you can—even if you need some form of assistance. Be sure to set realistic expectations for yourself, though.

OVERCOMING OBSTACLES

If you are:

- living alone, plan to share a weekly meal with a friend or neighbor.

- finding it difficult to get to the store, ask the local church, temple, or senior center for help, or use your grocery store's delivery service.

- taking medications, associate your meds with a regular daily activity so you won't miss a dose (for example, take a pill when you brush your teeth or with a certain meal).

- dealing with pain or lessened mobility, do things in stages. It may take several hours to complete a chore, but that's okay. Try using household objects as free weights to increase your strength and flexibility.

- **Manage your weight.** If you are overweight or obese, work with your healthcare provider to create a weight-loss plan that's right for you. Losing weight will lessen extra strain on your heart and reduce your risk of heart attack and stroke. On the other hand, if you are underweight, talk with your healthcare provider because being too thin can also put you at risk.

- **Monitor your heart health and follow through.** Stay vigilant and keep up with your healthcare appointments. Don't procrastinate—follow the recommendations of your doctor, and stick to your lifestyle "prescriptions" as carefully as you do to your medication regimen.

- **Maintain good communication with your doctors.** Partner with your healthcare providers and share information. Don't hold back because you are reluctant, afraid, or embarrassed. Ask for help if you need it; be sure you understand your options if you need treatment, and expect clear answers to your questions.

eating for a healthy heart

Good nutrition is one of the cornerstones of a healthy lifestyle at any age, promoting better heart health and vitality. As you get older, your body needs less food as your metabolism slows down—and even less if your mobility is reduced—but it's still important to feed your body well so it gets the nutrients it needs. The foods you choose are as vital as the pills you may take to care for your health.

Studies show that **diet has a profound effect on overall well-being.** Failing energy, decreased resistance to infection, greater risk for disease, and slower mental functioning are not necessarily "normal" effects of aging; in reality they may be the results of a diet that does not provide sufficient levels of essential nutrients. The key to eating healthy is to consistently make good choices from a wide variety of nutritious foods.

Healthy Food, Healthy Body

In general, you'll benefit most from eating more vegetables and fruits, adequate protein, and less sodium and harmful saturated and trans fats. You should limit high-calorie foods that provide little nutritional value, such as desserts, sodas, and fried foods, and concentrate on nutrient-dense foods that offer high nutritional value per calorie, such as fruits and vegetables, whole grains, fat-free and low-fat dairy products, fish, and lean poultry and meats. Be sure also to eat fiber-rich foods and drink liquids—both help with digestion and keep you hydrated.

Does all this mean you have to give up eating your favorite pie forever? No! Keep in mind that it's your overall eating plan that counts the most, not the occasional splurge. Once you set your mind to think of favorite high-calorie/nutrition-poor foods as special treats to enjoy every now and then, those foods will become the exceptions rather than the rule in your diet.

To get the most nutrition from your food, focus on:

- **A variety of vegetables and fruits.** For the widest range of nutrients, including vitamins and minerals, eat many different types and colors of vegetables and fruits, especially the deeply colored ones, such as spinach, carrots, kale, berries, apricots, and mangoes. They also are an excellent source of fiber, which can help your digestion. Based on a 2,000-calorie diet, you should aim to eat about five servings of vegetables and four servings of fruit each day. To help you reach that amount, you could include fruit as part of your breakfast routine, add salad greens and an apple to your lunch, snack on a handful of dried fruit in the afternoon, and enjoy vegetable side dishes with your dinner.

- **Whole-grain and high-fiber foods.** For another great source of dietary fiber, eat whole grains, which help reduce your risk for heart disease by keeping LDL cholesterol levels lower. Whole grains are much more nutritious than refined grains, so try brown rice and products that list a whole grain first on the ingredients label. Some common ones are corn or whole-grain cereals and whole-wheat or whole-grain breads and pastas. In general, women over 70 should aim for about 21 grams every day. For example, you could get off to a good start with a bowl of bran flakes and a medium banana for breakfast. Other fiber-rich foods include legumes such as kidney beans, pinto beans, chickpeas, and lentils, as well as fresh and dried fruits.

- **Fat-free and low-fat dairy products.** As you get older, it's important to include adequate amounts of calcium-rich foods in your diet because calcium can reduce the loss of minerals from bones and slow the development of osteoporosis. Try to eat enough fat-free or low-fat dairy foods, such as milk, cheeses, and yogurt, to reach a total of about 1,200 mg of calcium each day. For example, a cup of yogurt contains about 450 mg, a 3-ounce slice of fat-free cheese contains about 350 mg, and an 8-ounce glass of fat-free milk has about 300 mg of calcium. Eight ounces of calcium-fortified orange juice can supply an additional 110 mg of calcium. As you get older, the ability to absorb calcium declines, so you may need more vitamin D to help your body absorb the calcium you eat. Fortified milk products and breakfast cereals are good sources of vitamin D, as is exposure to sunlight.

- **Fish rich in omega-3 fatty acids.** The protective benefits of eating fish rich in omega-3 fatty acids include lowering blood pressure and LDL cholesterol levels. Omega-3 fats also can reduce blood clotting and the risk of heart arrhythmias. Studies have shown that omega-3 fatty acids may protect women who have already suffered a cardiac event from experiencing a second one. Eating about 6 ounces of cooked oil-rich fish per week may also help modulate inflammatory diseases, such as rheumatoid arthritis; improve insulin sensitivity; and slow down deteriorating eyesight. Omega-3 fats from fish also have been linked to lessening mental deterioration from dementia, Alzheimer's, and other conditions. Good sources of omega-3 fats are salmon, tuna, trout, sardines, and herring. Canned salmon or sardines, both with bones, are also good sources of calcium and protein.

american heart association
complete guide to women's heart health

- **Lean poultry and meats.** Protein remains an important part of good nutrition in your 70s. It provides essential nutrients, such as iron, that can be depleted by medications or that are not absorbed well by your body, and it helps your body rebuild and recuperate from illnesses or surgeries. Aim for about 46 grams of protein a day. Choose lean cuts such as chicken or turkey breast, sirloin, and pork tenderloin, for example. If you have high blood cholesterol, keep your intake of meats and poultry to 5 ounces (cooked) or less a day, making up the difference with vegetarian options, legumes, and dairy foods as needed. For example, you could have one scrambled egg white (4 grams), a sandwich made with whole-wheat bread and three slices of turkey breast (6 grams), a cup of yogurt for a snack (13 grams), and a burger made with 95 percent fat-free ground beef (4 ounces raw weight; 22 grams) to keep your saturated fat and cholesterol down and your protein intake up.

- **Legumes, nuts, and seeds.** Eating plenty of beans, lentils, chickpeas, and other legumes, such as peanuts, will give you more protein and fiber with less saturated fat and cholesterol than a meat-based diet. Nuts and seeds provide protein and heart-healthy unsaturated fats, which can help reduce LDL cholesterol and blood pressure. Unsalted nuts are good as snacks when eaten in moderation and as toppings on cereals, yogurt, stir-fries, and salads.

- **Healthy unsaturated oils and fats.** Fat is needed in your diet, but it's the type of fat consumed that makes the difference to your heart health. The "bad fats"—saturated and trans fats—increase your LDL cholesterol and your risk for heart disease. On the other hand, the "better fats"—unsaturated fats, such as monounsaturated and polyunsaturated—found in oils, nuts, fish, and avocado help increase HDL cholesterol and reduce your risk of heart disease and stroke. All fats, however, are high in calories, so choose wisely. For example, you'll get more nutritional benefit if you spend your fat calories on healthy oils in salad dressings or about 1½ ounces of walnuts four to five times a week instead of on unhealthy shortening or stick margarine in high-calorie cakes or cookies. If you are losing weight but don't want to be, be sure you are not unnecessarily restricting wholesome but higher-fat foods.

In addition to knowing what foods to include in your diet, it's important to know what to limit. To help you gauge how certain foods fit into your eating plan, use these guidelines as you make your food choices.

- **Aim to limit sodium to less than 1,500 mg a day.** Older women, especially African Americans and women with high blood pressure, need less than the 2,300 mg recommended for healthy younger adults.

- **Aim to limit cholesterol to less than 300 mg each day.v**

- **Aim to limit saturated and trans fats as much as possible.** Try to be sure that your intake of these harmful fats does not reach an unhealthy proportion of your daily calorie intake.

IF YOU USUALLY EAT THIS MANY CALORIES EACH DAY					
	1,200	**1,500**	**1,800**	**2,000**	**2,500**
Keep **saturated fat** to less than	9 grams	11 grams	13 grams	15 grams	19 grams
Keep **trans fat** to less than	1 gram	1.5 gram	2 grams	2 grams	2.5 grams

Because high blood pressure is so common in older women, it's important to keep the sodium (salt) in your diet to a minimum. In general, the more salt you eat, the higher your blood pressure. Since most of the sodium you eat actually comes from processed foods rather than from the salt you add during cooking or at the table, be sure to read the nutritional labels on food packages in the grocery stores and choose the lower-sodium options. In addition to cutting back on sodium, try to eat more foods that contain potassium, which helps counterbalance the effects of sodium on blood pressure. Bananas, cantaloupe, yogurt, orange juice, and potatoes are all excellent sources of potassium.

The aging process negatively affects your ability to absorb and use various nutrients. Your absorption of calcium and vitamin D, both important for good bone health, typically decreases with age, which in turn leaves you more vulnerable to osteoporosis and bone fractures. Other common deficiencies include magnesium, vitamin B_{12}, and vitamin C. You may need to add to your diet by eating fortified foods or taking supplements, but every woman's body is different and nutritional needs vary. Talk with your doctor to decide which nutrients your body may be lacking and the best ways to supplement your diet.

Dehydration also can become a problem as you get older. Your body becomes less able to detect thirst, so you may not realize you are thirsty. Be sure to include plenty of water and other fluids with your meals and throughout the day. Some healthy choices are vegetables, fruits, juices, fat-free milk, low-fat buttermilk, fat-free and low-fat yogurt drinks, low-sodium soups, and decaffeinated coffee and teas.

Overcoming Barriers to Eating Well

By your 70s, you may have encountered some mental or physical obstacles that interfere with your ability to eat well. If you live alone, mealtimes may be difficult or depressing. Cooking can become a burden. Limited income, difficulty getting out to shop, or physical problems with chewing or swallowing also can present challenges. Taste buds become less sensitive with age, and some medications and illnesses also change the way food tastes, which can make eating less appealing. The demands of following special or restricted diets as well as changes in your mental state, such as depression, can affect your interest in eating as well.

If you are facing any of these barriers, you may settle into the habit of eating packaged foods such as frozen dinners, canned foods, and lunch meats because they are quick and easy. If so, be mindful that many of these foods are high in calories, saturated fat, and sodium and may offer little nutritional value. Or you may find you gradually eat less as your interest in food declines. If you start to lose weight without making any intentional effort to do so, talk with your doctor and identify the cause. Being underweight can make you more prone to infection and leave you with low muscle mass, leading to increased risk of osteoporosis, anemia, and other health problems.

Whatever the reason, if you have lost interest in eating a balanced diet, you are depriving your body of the nutrients it needs to be healthy and strong. Here are some ideas to make eating more satisfying and healthful:

- **Eat with someone** whose company you enjoy as often as you can.

- Try new recipes or different herbs, spices, or salt-free seasoning blends to **spark your interest in food.**

- **Keep an eating area cleared and set.** For a special touch, add a nice cloth, pretty tableware, and a flower in a vase to create a positive environment.

- **Eat several light meals a day** instead of three heavier meals.

- **Tempt your taste buds** with smaller portions of several foods at one meal.

- Give yourself permission to snack, but **snack healthy.** Keep nutritious finger foods on hand, such as fat-free cheese sticks, fruit, and whole-grain crackers.

- **Don't feel bound by convention:** try having a bowl of low-sodium broth with chickpeas for breakfast, then end the day with a bowl of oatmeal, topped with yogurt, fruit, and nuts.

- **Focus on quality.** It's a better use of your calorie quota to treat yourself to one special cookie that you really enjoy than to eat three mediocre ones.

- To **keep trips to the store to a minimum,** buy enough of your favorite fresh, packaged, canned, and frozen foods to last at least a week.

- **Carefully read the nutrition facts panels on packaged food labels.** Many health-conscious products are available now, but you may have to look for them. Pay less attention to the advertising on the front of the packaging and more attention to the actual nutrition facts on the back or side. It's definitely worth the time because levels of nutrients can vary a lot between similar products. For example, one brand of frozen chicken entrée can contain twice as much fat and sodium as another.

- **Buy fruits and vegetables in the form that works best for you**—fresh, frozen, or canned. Frozen and canned fruits and vegetables are packed just after being harvested, at the height of their nutritional value. Buy canned fruit packed in water or juice rather than syrup and look for frozen and canned vegetables with no or very little sodium added.

- **Eat fruits and vegetables in a variety of colors.** For example, incorporate a dark green vegetable and a bright orange or red vegetable or fruit into each day's meals and snacks. They not only look attractive but also are nutritious.

- **Think of meat as a side dish** so that you have room to add more vegetables, fruits, and grains to your meals. Instead of meat taking up half the plate, it should cover about a quarter of it, with a grain on another quarter, and colorful vegetables or fruit on the other half.

- **Plan meals so you can shop and cook once,** then enjoy the results several times during the week or make options that freeze well so you can keep leftovers for later use. You might also try "repurposing" the leftovers—for instance, chopping an extra baked chicken breast half and adding it to a soup, salad, or stir-fry.

- If the cost of healthy food is a challenge for you, **investigate the nutrition programs available in your area.** Many states offer assistance to eligible seniors through coupon books or a meal delivery service.

- **Shop with a friend or relative and buy in bulk to cut food costs.** You'll enjoy the company and share in the savings, too.

maintaining an active lifestyle

Contrary to the previously held idea that people's hearts just wear out as they get older, science has shown that by keeping your heart "primed" with regular aerobic exercise, you'll improve your overall fitness and stamina—and lessen the effects of age-related changes in your cardiovascular system. Simply put, **being physically active on a regular basis can help you stay mobile and independent.**

Why Exercise Is So Important to Your Heart

Although it's true that your body's capacity for strenuous exercise declines with age, study after study confirms that **getting blood pumping with exercise confers a wide range of physical and mental benefits, especially for seniors.** As scientists learn more about the mechanics of aging, they are starting to understand better how subtle internal changes affect an individual's experience of getting older.

As described in the introduction to this chapter your cardiovascular system undergoes changes that help it adapt as your body ages. Arteries stiffen and become less elastic, and the heart enlarges as it works harder to pump blood effectively. When you exert yourself physically, your heart beats even faster and harder to provide a sufficient amount of oxygen to the cells in your body. The structural changes within the heart that occur over time, in combination with functional changes that include decreased heart rate and weaker contractions, can make you feel more short of breath on exertion as the years pass.

Even if you have been inactive for some time, however, **your heart is remarkably resilient.** As is true for the other muscles in your body, **exercising your heart will make it stronger.** And the stronger your heart is, the better able it will be to adapt to these age-related changes and improve your capacity for physical activity.

Being active throughout your 70s will:

- help you maintain a healthy weight

- reduce arterial stiffening

- lower blood pressure

- reduce levels of harmful LDL cholesterol and increase helpful HDL cholesterol

- help manage diabetes if you have it

- slow the rate of bone loss and counteract the effects of osteoporosis

- strengthen the heart muscle and increase cardiovascular capacity

- increase flexibility and balance, lessening the risk of falling

- reduce muscle pain

- improve circulation and increase the delivery of oxygen and nutrients to your body's cells

- prevent arrhythmia, such as atrial fibrillation

- improve mental functioning

- boost self-confidence and elevate mood

- delay the onset of frailty

Resisting the Spiral of Inactivity

Living a sedentary life can create a downward spiral of *in*activity. Once you become accustomed to sitting most of the day, it's harder to use joints and muscles that aren't used to movement. The effort it takes to walk or climb stairs then reinforces the idea that you can't do as much as before, which leads you to sit down again and avoid activity, feeding the spiral. That's why it's so important as you get older to resist the tendency to sit more and move less.

If you have been sedentary for some time, don't let fear or habit stop you from changing to a more active routine. Ask your doctor to help you determine an appropriate level of effort relative to your level of fitness, and what kind of exercise is best for you. For most women, walking is an easy way to get started. All you really need is a comfortable pair of shoes and a safe place to walk. Studies have shown that even the normal activities of daily living, such as housework or gardening, can increase heart rate enough to provide health benefits, as long as you put some exertion or elbow grease into them.

Find an Activity That Fits

If you are active now, keep up your usual routine. As time goes on, you can take it easier if you need to, but **don't stop moving. Listen to your body and do whatever fits your capabilities best.** (If you have an existing chronic condition, learn whether and how it affects your ability to be physically active.) Use your imagination, have fun, and get moving! On the other hand, if you haven't been active and aren't sure what to do to set yourself in motion, here are some ideas:

- **Join a fitness or community center that provides programs,** such as water aerobics, line-dancing classes, and yoga classes, targeted for seniors.

- **Check into the programs at your local city parks** that offer exercise classes for seniors.

- **Go to your local library or video rental store to look for exercise videos and DVDs** created for older women that are suitable for your activity level whether beginner, advanced, or somewhere in between. Try a variety of options—strength training, Pilates, yoga, tai chi—so you can to determine what suits your physical capabilities and what you enjoy most.

- **Go bowling, square dancing, or ballroom dancing.**

- **Go for nature walks or bird-watching.**

- **Find a walking buddy** and meet for a daily walk around the neighborhood, your favorite shopping mall, or the park.

- **Get competitive.** Enjoy a round of golf, or invite some neighbors over for a game of badminton or horseshoes.

How Much Is Enough?

How much exercise should you be doing? Talk with your doctor to determine what's right for you, but the recommendations for aerobic exercise for older women are the same as for younger women, and so are the benefits. **Aim for at least 150 minutes** (2 hours and 30 minutes) **of moderate-intensity aerobic activity a week, or 75 minutes** (1 hour and 15 minutes) **of vigorous-intensity aerobic activity,** or an equivalent combination of moderate and vigorous. **You can break the goal into increments of at least 10 minutes of aerobic activity,** such as walking the dog, preferably spread through the week. (Even something as simple as parking your car across the parking lot instead of in front of your destination is helpful.) To determine whether an activity counts as moderate or vigorous, think in terms of a 10-point scale, with 10 being the most strenuous. If you would rank the activity as a 5 or 6 and it causes noticeable increases in your heart rate and breathing, it would be a moderate activity. If you would rate it about 7 or 8 and you have *significant* increases in heart rate and breathing, that would be a strenuous activity. These results will depend, however, on your overall fitness level.

In addition to aerobic activity, you should do resistance exercises at least twice a week on days that aren't consecutive. These activities strengthen the major muscles of your body by working them against a force or weight. The level of resistance should be demanding enough to allow for only about ten to fifteen repetitions of each exercise. Also remember to stretch before a workout and include movements that maintain or increase your flexibility. Activities that improve your balance, such as tai chi or dancing, also help reduce the risk of falls.

Your goal is to **make physical activity a routine part of your life.** To do this, create an exercise plan that includes both aerobic and resistance exercise at the appropriate intensity level. Try to find an approach that is comfortable for you and includes activities you enjoy. If you are not used to being active, start slow and easy, and then gradually increase your level of activity. Even at a slower pace, you'll still be benefiting from your efforts, regardless of how long it takes you to work up to the recommended goals. If you are already fit and active, exercising longer or more often will further improve your fitness level—and help reduce your risk for disease. Whether you are an exercise veteran or a novice, be sure to monitor your progress as you go and reassess your exercise routine so that it is in line with your current abilities and health status. (See Appendix C for an activity diary.)

If you have limitations because of a medical condition, you can still work up to a level of activity that is appropriate for you. Carefully choose an activity that does not jeopardize your safety, even if that means using a cane or walker, getting assistance from a companion, or exercising from a chair. Remember that **any exercise is better than no exercise at all.**

Staying motivated to exercise can be difficult at any age, but being older can make it even harder. Ask yourself if your attitude is getting in your way. If you associate exercise with negative experiences and thoughts, try to let go of them and instead concentrate on all the ways being active will improve your physical *and* mental well-being. Research shows that physical activity boosts mental fitness and can reduce the effects of depression. Being active can help you feel happier and more confident, and visualizing yourself as a mobile, fit, and active woman will help motivate you to get moving and stay moving.

managing your weight

Being a healthy weight in your 70s is as important to your health as it's ever been. If you are overweight or obese, you are adding to the strain on your older heart. **Carrying extra pounds increases the heart's workload and makes you more vulnerable to higher blood pressure, diabetes, and heart disease and heart attack.** Losing extra weight will reduce those risks. For example, by losing 20 pounds, you could lower your blood pressure by 5 to 20 mmHg.

With every passing year, your body composition shifts a little at a time. Muscle mass decreases, and fat tissue increases. Since muscle requires more energy than fat, the less muscle tissue overall, the fewer calories your body needs for everyday metabolic functions. If you haven't adjusted how you eat as you've gotten older, you most likely have gained weight, although some women do begin to lose too much weight in their later years. The good news in either circumstance is that by making some changes to your diet and adding more physical activity, you can gain control over your weight. Because maximizing the nutritional value of what you eat is so important in your 70s, however, achieving and maintaining a healthy weight involves more than just watching calories. **It's not only the quantity but also the quality of what you eat that matters.**

Reaching a Healthy Weight Safely

Science has shown that the simple formula of **calories in = calories out is the best approach to maintaining your weight.** In other words, to stay at your current weight, you need to balance how much you eat with how much energy you burn.

To assess your calorie intake, write down everything you eat and drink for a week. (You can use the food diary at the end of Appendix C.) At the end of the week, calculate your average daily calorie count. Refer to the box on page 253 to determine the number of calories you can eat each day to maintain your current weight. Compare that number with your actual daily calorie average. If your actual daily calorie intake is more than what you need to maintain your weight, you will gradually gain weight. If you need to lose weight, you will need to find ways to eat fewer calories on average and move more.

Use your food diary to identify the sources of extra calories. Look for patterns, such as high-calorie foods you eat often and triggers for overeating. Then find ways to substitute a lower-calorie alternative or defuse the triggers. For example, if you eat dessert every night, swap the usual bowl of ice cream for a colorful piece of sweet, juicy fruit. If you keep cookies or candy in the house for grandchildren or in case company drops by, keep those treats where you won't be as tempted to indulge when you're by yourself. The "they're for company" foods can sabotage your best efforts to eat wisely.

If you are overweight, here are some weight management techniques you can use to start losing those extra pounds:

- **Serve yourself smaller portions** of high-calorie, low-nutrient foods.

- **Eat three-quarters of the amount of food you currently eat.**

- **Satisfy cravings with a small tidbit of high-quality dark chocolate,** for example, rather than an entire candy bar.

- **Learn to recognize appropriate portion sizes.** For example, a single serving of pasta should be about half a cup, or the size of a baseball.

- **Find lower-calorie substitutes for the foods you eat regularly.** Replace whole milk with fat-free milk or fat-free half-and-half, and enjoy fruit sorbet or a homemade fruit smoothie instead of regular ice cream for dessert.

- **Choose a variety of different types and colors of vegetables and fruits** to replace higher-calorie foods.

- **Use heart-healthy sources of unsaturated fat,** such as canola and olive oils, nuts, and avocados, **sparingly** since they are high in calories.

- **Ask yourself before you eat a certain treat if it is worth "spending" your calorie allotment on.** If so, enjoy it for the moment, but remember to cut back on something else later to keep your calorie count balanced.

- **Be wary of soft drinks and packaged baked goods that provide empty calories** but very few if any nutrients.

- **Keep small amounts of nutritious snacks available to nibble on** throughout the day, both to stave off hunger and keep your metabolism from hitting highs and lows. Examples include a small handful of nuts (no more than 1½ ounces four to five days per week), fresh or dried fruit, and fat-free cheeses.

- **Read the nutrition facts on labels** (not the marketing information on the front) of frozen or packaged dinners **and choose the healthier options.** Many packaged foods are high in fats, sodium, and calories.

- **Set up a routine to get up and moving for 30 to 60 minutes a day.**

The key to successful weight management is balancing your intake of food with your level of activity. Although counting calories and portion control are keys to controlling your weight, **good nutrition should be your top priority.** If you make good choices every day, your efforts will add up to a healthier weight and a healthier heart.

managing your health care

If you are a woman in your 70s, **your risk for heart disease and heart attack is at least as great as that of a man—perhaps more so.** In 2004, 454,613 women died of cardiovascular disease, compared with 409,867 men. In the last 25 years, the number of deaths has declined for both males and females, but since 1984, more females than males have died of cardiovascular disease. These statistics have raised questions about the differences between men and women and how those differences affect their risks, health care, and outcomes.

New research may explain why heart disease looks different in women than in men. In general, extra weight on women tends to be distributed in many areas of their bodies, whereas men tend to carry most of their extra weight in their abdomen. This difference in distribution of body fat may be mirrored in how arterial plaque collects. Plaque in men develops in arteries as large blockages in one or two areas; researchers have found evidence that plaque in women may be spread evenly throughout the smaller coronary arteries. Both types of plaque obstruct the flow of blood and oxygen, but tests such as angiograms are not designed to find blockages in the smaller arteries. This makes diagnosis much more difficult and may account for many cases of unrecognized heart disease in women; if left untreated, the heart disease can lead to a full-blown heart attack.

The average age for women to have a first heart attack is 70. As it is for men, women's most common heart attack symptom is chest pain or discomfort. **Women, however, are somewhat more likely to experience some of the other common symptoms, particularly shortness of breath, nausea or vomiting, and back or jaw pain.**

Because many women are not aware of their risk or are afraid of "making a fuss," they wait too long to get help. **If you experience unexpected chest pain that doesn't go away in a few minutes or other signs of a heart attack, call 9-1-1, and don't wait more than five minutes to take action.** (For more information on the warning signs of heart attack and stroke, see Appendix E.)

If you have angina and take nitroglycerin tablets, call 9-1-1 if your symptoms worsen or are not relieved after three tablets. If you notice that your angina is more frequent or requires the maximum dose of nitroglycerin, be sure to follow up with your healthcare provider.

Partner with Your Healthcare Team

It shouldn't take an emergency, of course, to get you to see your doctor. **It's important to schedule regular checkups with your healthcare provider team to watch for potential problems and monitor and address the risk factors you may already have.** Using the latest information available, you and your doctors can work together to either prevent heart disease or recognize it early if it develops—and stop it from worsening. With the right changes in your lifestyle and medical treatment, it may be possible to prevent further development of coronary artery disease.

Researchers are working to close the gender gap in health care and develop new technologies that will provide better imaging and diagnostic tools for women. These advances will help your doctor do a better job of keeping you and your heart healthy. You need to do your part, too, though. **It's really up to you to follow through and be a good steward of your own heart health.**

Although you may be tempted to put off visits to your doctor until something hurts so much you can't ignore it, keep in mind that it's important to be proactive where your health is concerned. Don't let fear of getting bad news or reluctance to undergo testing make you procrastinate. Schedule regular doctor visits and be sure you find out the numbers for your blood pressure, cholesterol, glucose levels, and weight.

Good communication between patient and doctor is key to effective medical care. You are a critical part of the team, and your collaboration is essential. If you feel uncomfortable with your doctor and her or his staff, find other medical professionals who earn your confidence and listen carefully to you. Don't worry more about insulting your doctor than you do about meeting your health needs. It's important to find a doctor you can trust and communicate with openly and honestly. Remember that you are your own best advocate.

As part of an effective partnership, **you should take a written list of symptoms, questions, and concerns to your appointments so that your doctor** will have all the needed facts and you will remember everything you need to discuss while there. Likewise, write down the answers to your questions, as well as other instructions from your doctor, before you leave the office. Many healthcare providers also offer printed health information that you can take home. (For more guidance on how to get the most from your healthcare partners, see Appendix B.)

The results of the Women's Health Study suggest that **taking aspirin every day can help women in their 70s prevent both heart attack and stroke.** Be sure to discuss the best strategy for your health with your healthcare provider, assess your risk, and weigh the potential benefits of aspirin against any possible problems it may cause, such as gastrointestinal bleeding. (For more information, see the special section called "Aspirin Therapy: What Is Recommended?" on page 175.)

Managing Risk Factors in Your 70s

By age 70, most women are already working to manage at least one of the major risk factors for heart disease. If you are in that position, you may want to **consider adding a cardiologist to your healthcare team.** Having a risk factor increases your chances of developing heart disease or having a heart attack, but it does not guarantee that either will occur. Keep in mind that it's *never* too late to take action to control, or limit the effects of, your risk factors. The following section discusses the major risk factors that you are most likely to face in your 70s.

HIGH BLOOD PRESSURE
Reducing your blood pressure even a little bit can dramatically improve your health and reduce your risk of coronary artery disease and stroke.

High blood pressure can also increase the loss of calcium that leads to osteoporosis. A combination of lifestyle changes and medications can keep your blood pressure under control, which is an important goal at any age.

UNHEALTHY CHOLESTEROL LEVELS AND TRIGLYCERIDES

Although a high level of LDL cholesterol is considered a serious risk factor for heart disease, growing evidence shows that the best predictor of your risk as an older woman is the level of HDL cholesterol. HDL cholesterol appears to protect against the artery-clogging plaque that LDL cholesterol deposits. If your HDL levels are low, you are at increased risk for developing coronary artery disease. Be sure that you are given a complete profile of your total LDL and HDL cholesterol levels. Again, the most effective treatment is a combination of lifestyle changes and medications.

High levels of triglycerides, another type of blood fat, also increase your risk for heart disease and are associated with high LDL cholesterol, low HDL cholesterol, and obesity. Calories not used immediately are converted into triglycerides, which are then transported to fat cells to be stored. When your triglyceride level is too high, it can increase blood viscosity (or thickness), making it harder for blood to flow freely. High triglycerides significantly increase your risk of heart attack, even if your blood cholesterol levels are normal. The first approach to treatment for high triglycerides is lifestyle change: lose weight if needed, reduce your intake of saturated and trans fats and dietary cholesterol, avoid alcohol, eat a balanced diet, and make regular physical activity part of your routine. If your triglycerides are very high or you have family history that puts you at additional risk, your doctor may recommend more aggressive treatment such as medication as well.

PHYSICAL INACTIVITY

In addition to the associated risk of cardiovascular disease, sedentary behavior, such as hours spent watching television, can contribute to obesity and the risk of type 2 diabetes. Conversely, more physical activity will reduce the effects of risk factors such as high blood pressure and LDL cholesterol and will help control existing diabetes.

DIABETES

Diabetes tends to develop with age, and for women it is a particularly potent risk factor for heart disease. Once you have diabetes, your risk of developing coronary heart disease increases three to seven times. That's why it's so important to have your blood glucose level checked as often as your healthcare provider recommends and to keep up the lifestyle habits that can prevent both diabetes and other risk factors: eating for good nutrition and staying physically active. If you already have diabetes, be sure to follow your doctor's recommendations—you can still significantly reduce your risk for heart disease by keeping your blood sugar levels under control.

METABOLIC SYNDROME

Diabetes is also associated with *metabolic syndrome,* a cluster of risk factors that greatly increases your risk for cardiovascular disease. If you have three or more of these conditions, you are considered to have metabolic syndrome:

- Waist measurement equal to or greater than 35 inches

- Triglyceride level of 150 mg/dL or higher

- HDL cholesterol less than 50 mg/dL

- Systolic blood pressure of 130 mmHg or higher

- Diastolic blood pressure of 85 mmHg or higher

- Fasting glucose reading of 100 mg/dL or higher

. . .

While your senior years definitely carry increased risk for heart disease and heart attack, the medical community has made great strides in diagnosing and treating these conditions, especially in women. If you are living with heart disease now or managing risk factors, your participation in your own health care is the critical link between your doctor's recommendations and the most effective outcome.

checklist for achieving heart health in your 70s and beyond

✓ **Make eating well a priority.**

✓ **Stay as physically active as you can.**

✓ **Develop a plan** to eat for good nutrition and add regular exercise to your life.

✓ **Follow the plan** and modify it if necessary.

✓ **Keep your weight at a healthy level** by balancing your food intake with your level of activity. Cut back on less nutritious foods if you need to lose weight.

✓ **Partner with a network of trusted healthcare professionals.**

✓ **Get regular health checkups and communicate openly with your healthcare providers.**

✓ **Monitor your risk factors**—especially elevated blood pressure, unhealthy cholesterol levels, diabetes, physical inactivity, and overweight and obesity.

✓ **Follow your doctor's recommendations** for managing risk factors or existing heart disease.

✓ **Take medications as prescribed** by your healthcare professionals.

✓ **Know the warning signs of heart attack and stroke.**

part three

health care
for your
heart

CHAPTER 9

common tests

As part of your regular health checkups, you will most likely undergo some tests to determine how your heart is functioning.

Just the word *test* makes many people uncomfortable or nervous. Understanding why these tests are so valuable and how they contribute to an accurate diagnosis may help dispel some of your fear and anxiety. Feel free to share with your healthcare providers any questions, uncertainties, or apprehensions you may have about these tests.

screening tests

Most screening tests, such as drawing blood for testing, are conducted in your doctor's office as part of your physical examination. Depending on the results of these preliminary screenings, your doctor may send you for further testing to pinpoint the cause for an abnormal finding.

A heart-related physical examination should include measurement of your heart rate, heart rhythm, pulse at various places on your body, and blood pressure. Your doctor will also look for signs of swelling (called edema), especially in your legs and ankles, and listen to your heart and lungs with a stethoscope, a process called auscultation. These simple steps actually tell your doctor quite a lot about your heart function, blood flow, and the condition of your circulatory system. Your doctor also will check the blood vessels at the back of your eyes, since any damage visible there may signal similar damage occurring in vessels elsewhere in your body.

In addition to the recommended tests that measure levels of blood pressure, cholesterol, and glucose, your doctor may request more specific blood tests that provide important information about your general health. Laboratory analyses of your blood, including a complete blood count, expanded lipid profile, and oxygen content, can identify infection, as well as many other indicators of how well your body is functioning. The results of these tests may lead to a quick diagnosis or tell your doctor whether to proceed with further testing.

diagnostic tests

If your screening tests show some abnormality or you are experiencing symptoms of heart disease, your doctor may schedule a diagnostic test. These tests are used to both rule out possible disorders and pinpoint the correct cause of your symptoms. Most tests used in the early stages of diagnosing heart-related conditions are noninvasive and painless.

Your doctor chooses which (and how many) tests to perform on the basis of several considerations, including your existing risk factors, history of heart problems, current symptoms, and your doctor's interpretation of how these factors intersect. Typically the simplest, least invasive tests are used first, graduating to the more complicated and invasive tests only as necessary.

Electrocardiography is the first and most basic method used to determine the general condition of your heart. An electrocardiogram (referred to as an ECG or EKG) creates a graphic record of the heart's electrical impulses. These recordings can be clinical (measured in a doctor's office) or ambulatory (measured during your normal activities). This very common and painless test shows whether your heart rate and rhythm are normal, and it can identify inadequate blood flow to the heart muscle (ischemia), possible heart damage, and other cardiac problems. To record an ECG, the technician will attach several wires, or leads, to your chest and sometimes your arms and legs as well. As you lie still, each lead records the same electrical impulse but from a different position in relation to your heart. A twelve-lead ECG, for example, allows your doctor to view twelve different recordings at the same time. For an ambulatory reading, you may be asked to wear either a portable 24-hour Holter monitor to record your heart's impulses as you go about your daily routine or a recorder that you can turn on when you feel an event occurring. The ECG readings can then be transmitted for analysis by attaching the recorder directly to a telephone receiver.

Exercise stress tests (also called treadmill tests) demonstrate how well your heart can handle physical exertion by recording ECG readings during exercise. If you are scheduled for a stress test, you'll probably be asked to avoid strenuous activity on the day of the test and eat no food for two to three hours beforehand. Dress comfortably in clothes you can exercise in, and wear walking shoes. A technician will attach ECG leads to your chest and you will be asked to walk in place on a treadmill. After a few minutes, the difficulty of the exercise will gradually increase as the technician increases the speed and/or tilt of the treadmill. As your body works harder to keep pace with the treadmill, it requires more oxygen, so your heart must pump more blood. During the test, technicians will monitor your ECG readings, heart rate, breathing, and blood pressure, and how tired you feel throughout the test.

A stress test can show whether the blood supply is reduced in the coronary arteries and can also help your doctor know what level of exercise is safe for you. Stress testing poses very little risk for healthy women, but medical professionals should be present in case something unusual happens during the test. Your doctor may recommend an exercise stress test to:

- Diagnose a possible heart-related cause of symptoms such as chest pain, shortness of breath, or lightheadedness.

- Diagnose coronary artery disease.

- Check the effectiveness of procedures done to improve coronary artery circulation in patients with existing coronary artery disease.

- Predict risk of dangerous heart-related conditions such as a heart attack.

If you experience palpitations or chest pain during the test, tell the doctor or technician immediately. Don't be alarmed until the results of your test have been reviewed by your doctor. **It's not uncommon for exercise stress tests to result in false-positive readings, particularly in women.**

Thallium stress tests use nuclear scanning to show how well blood flows to the heart muscle and are usually performed with an exercise stress test on a treadmill or stationary bicycle. When you reach your maximum level of exercise, a small amount of the radioisotope thallium is injected into a vein. The thallium mixes with your blood and enters the heart muscle cells, leaving a flow pattern that can be imaged and recorded. If part of your heart muscle isn't receiving a normal blood supply, less thallium will appear in those heart muscle cells. The images taken after exercise show the blood flow that occurred during exercise. You may be asked to lie quietly for two to three hours so another series of images can be taken to show blood flow to the heart muscle during rest for comparison.

Physicians use thallium stress tests to determine causes of chest pain, assess levels of coronary artery blockage, and identify damaged heart muscle after a heart attack. If the pattern of thallium is normal during both exercise and rest, blood flow through your coronary arteries is normal. If the test shows that blood flow is normal during rest but not during exercise, the heart isn't getting enough blood when it must work harder than normal. This may be due to a blockage in one or more coronary arteries. If the test is abnormal during both exercise and rest, there's limited blood flow to that part of the heart at all times. If no thallium is seen in some part of the heart muscle, the cells in this part of the heart have died because of a prior heart attack. Thallium tests also are used to gauge the effectiveness of cardiac procedures done to improve circulation in coronary arteries.

If you are unable to exercise hard enough for a stress test, doctors can use drugs to induce a similar level of stress to your cardiovascular system. Medications such as dipyridamole or dobutamine are injected to dilate the coronary arteries and increase blood flow. If an artery is blocked, it will not expand as expected during the test, and the obstruction can be identified with a thallium scan.

american heart association
complete guide to women's heart health

Echocardiography uses ultrasound (high-frequency sound waves) to show the shape, texture, and movement of the heart's walls and valves. The recordings also show the size of the heart chambers and how well they're functioning. This painless test poses no risk and will be familiar if you had ultrasound pictures taken of your baby while you were pregnant. A **stress echocardiogram** is recorded before and during or immediately after some form of physical stress, such as exercise on a stationary bicycle or treadmill. This type of echocardiography is especially useful in establishing whether shortness of breath is caused by coronary artery disease, heart failure, or valvular heart disease, and it may be more accurate in women than an ECG stress test. For even more defined imaging of the heart and its structures, your doctor may suggest a **transesophageal echocardiogram** (TEE). The esophagus is right behind the heart, so TEE images can deliver very clear pictures and provide crucial information for an accurate diagnosis. Because this test involves passing a tube with a transducer at the end through the throat and into the esophagus, you will be sedated and given a local anesthetic for the procedure. **Doppler ultrasound** uses ultrasound imaging to measure the blood flow through arteries and veins, which helps identify blood vessels that may be narrowed.

Computed tomography (CT), including conventional, helical, and electron-beam ("ultrafast") forms, uses noninvasive X-ray technology to provide cross-sectional images of the chest, including the heart and blood vessels. You will be asked to lie on a table that is moved slowly through a large X-ray machine. CT scanning is useful in evaluating aortic disease, cardiac masses, and pericardial disease. **Electron-beam CT** can be used to measure the presence of calcium, specifically in the form of calcified plaque in the arteries. New research indicates that the more calcified plaque you have, the more likely you are to have coronary artery disease. The amount of calcium the scan detects is related to the amount of underlying coronary atherosclerosis and may help predict the likelihood of cardiac events such as heart attacks or the need for procedures such as coronary bypass surgery or angioplasty in the future. If no calcium is present, you may be at lower risk for future coronary events. **Positron emission tomography** (PET) combines tomographic imaging with radionuclide tracers to graphically demonstrate the heart's blood flow, structure, and cellular metabolism. Intense color on the test results shows diseased areas in tissues and organs. This imaging technique very accurately detects coronary artery disease and is also used to evaluate injury to the heart muscle. PET can distinguish between heart muscle that is not functioning properly but is still viable and muscle that has suffered permanent cell death. Patients with heart failure or who have had a heart attack are good candidates for PET.

Magnetic resonance imaging (MRI) uses radio waves and powerful magnets to provide images of inside the body. You will be asked to lie on a table that is moved into a large hollow chamber. A scanner receives radio waves from the areas of your body being scanned and processes the signals into computer-generated images. (If you tend to feel anxious in closed spaces, tell your healthcare provider; open MRI equipment is also available.) MRI images can show how well heart muscle is functioning, identify damage from a heart attack, and evaluate disease of the larger blood vessels such as the aorta. It is used to diagnose congenital heart disease, cardiomyopathy, congestive heart failure, and valve disease. **Magnetic resonance angiography (MRA)** combines the same technology with the injection of a contrast medium, or dye, to visualize and measure blood flow to the heart.

A more invasive procedure, **coronary angiography,** or cardiac catheterization, uses X-ray imaging to visualize arteries, veins, and chambers of the heart. The procedure is performed in the cardiac catheterization laboratory (you'll hear it referred to as the "cath lab") on either an inpatient or an outpatient basis. While you are lying on a table, the cardiologist will insert a catheter (a tiny flexible tube) into a blood vessel in your femoral artery in the groin area. The catheter is moved up through the arteries to the heart, where the tip is positioned either in the heart or at the beginning of the arteries supplying the heart, and a contrast dye is injected. (Most often the movement of the catheter itself is not felt, but occasionally a warm sensation or tingling is reported when the dye is released.) As the dye moves through the network of coronary arteries, its presence shows any blockages that are reducing blood flow. The images, or angiograms, can be recorded on video or in a sequential series.

Angiograms show narrowing in an artery or vessel. If during the procedure a blocked artery is discovered, your doctor may decide to do an

american heart association
complete guide to women's heart health

angioplasty to open the blockage and increase blood flow to help prevent a future heart attack (see page 224 for more information). Although any invasive procedure carries some risk, in most cases angiography is very safe and can provide crucial information in diagnosing heart disease or preventing heart attack. It is very useful in determining whether you need surgery, and the resulting images can act as a road map to guide your surgeon.

Angiography is quite effective in identifying obstructions of blood flow in the large main arteries. However, in some women plaque is distributed throughout smaller arteries, where it is more difficult to detect. It's also difficult to identify spasms in the arteries with standard tests. If you undergo angiography for chest pain or other symptoms of coronary artery disease but your angiogram seems clear, your doctor may order another type of test for a more definitive answer.

. . .

Despite the trepidation you might feel as you are undergoing various tests, remember that these advances in modern technology have provided the medical community with many valuable tools to help fight—and prevent—heart disease. Test results also help inform the decisions you and your healthcare team make about the prevention and treatment options that are best for you. Both screening and diagnostic tests provide specific, useful information that your doctors use in determining an accurate diagnosis.

COMMON SCREENING AND DIAGNOSTIC TESTS	POSSIBLE DIAGNOSIS
ECG, stress tests, Holter monitor and/or event recorder	Arrhythmia
ECG, blood tests, echocardiography, stress tests, nuclear scanning (CT and PET), coronary angiography	Coronary artery disease
Blood pressure tests, ankle-brachial index, ultrasound, angiography	Peripheral vascular disease
ECG, chest X-ray, stress tests, echocardiography, angiography, MRI, nuclear scanning (CT and PET), pulmonary function tests	Heart failure
ECG, chest X-ray, ultrasound, stress tests, angiography, MRI	Valve disease

common diagnoses and treatment options

Your doctor uses your test results in conjunction with what he or she knows about your symptoms, medical history, family history, and lifestyle habits to arrive at the best assessment of your situation. It is important to discuss the outcome of your clinical examination, lab work, and diagnostic tests with your healthcare providers. If the results are conclusive, your doctor will explain the cause of your symptoms and the initial diagnosis. Sometimes more investigation is needed to pinpoint a diagnosis, and you may be referred for further testing to find a definitive answer.

In this chapter, you'll find information on some of the most common heart-related diagnoses, including arrhythmias, coronary artery disease, peripheral vascular disease, heart failure, heart valve disorders, and congenital heart defects. You'll also read about common treatment options, which are described following each of the diagnoses. Be sure to discuss in detail with your doctors your diagnosis and the treatment options that are best for you.

arrhythmias

Arrhythmias are changes or abnormalities in the heart's natural rhythm. Almost everyone experiences some arrhythmia, perhaps an extra or a skipped beat now and then, or some minor palpitations caused by too much caffeine, stress, or even a decongestant. On the other hand, **some** arrhythmias can be severe and life threatening; the important thing is understanding what in the heart is creating the disturbance.

The rhythm of the heartbeat is controlled by electrical signals to the heart muscle sent via the sinoatrial node, your body's natural pacemaker. These electrical impulses trigger an intricate series of muscle contractions through the chambers of the heart. The alternating contraction and relaxation of the muscle moves blood from one chamber to the next, with the heart reacting as needed to messages sent by the brain or by hormones such as adrenaline, for example. When this process is disrupted by any number of causes, the rhythmic pace of your heart is also disturbed.

Bradycardia, a slower than normal heart rate, can result from a failure of the signal that tells your heart to deliver more blood or from damage to the sinoatrial node. Sinus bradycardia is defined as fewer than 60 beats per minute. In some cases, a slower heart rate causes no symptoms and is considered normal and benign. On the other hand, if you experience dizziness or shortness of breath with bradycardia, it could mean too little oxygen is being delivered to your body.

Tachycardia means your heart is beating too fast. Defined as any arrhythmia greater than 100 beats per minute, tachycardia can take several forms, which range from mild to severe and dangerous. There are two classifications of rapid heartbeat:

Supraventricular tachycardias originate above the ventricles in the atria. Conditions in this category include

- atrial tachycardia

- Wolff-Parkinson-White syndrome

- atrial flutter

- atrial fibrillation

Ventricular tachycardia originates in the ventricles themselves. If the sinoatrial node stops controlling the electrical signaling through the heart, the heart muscle will fail to contract properly, and heart rate increases. This most commonly occurs when heart disease is present. The most serious of arrhythmias, ventricular fibrillation, is an uncontrolled, very rapid heartbeat that can reach up to 300 beats per minute. This very fast beating is not effective, so the heart cannot pump enough blood to the brain and body. Ventricular fibrillation causes loss of consciousness and sudden death if not attended to immediately. If blood flow and oxygenation can be maintained with CPR (cardiopulmonary resuscitation) until the heart rhythm can be restored with an electric shock, it is possible to revive the person and reduce heart damage. That's why **it is important to learn bystander CPR and to know how to use an AED (automated external defibrillator).**

At the other end of the spectrum, many healthy women experience palpitations that are harmless, especially in the absence of underlying heart disease. For example, if you occasionally feel as if your heart is irregular or pounding, you may actually be experiencing the common arrhythmia called *premature ventricular contraction (PVC).* In this condition, your heart signals an early heartbeat but you typically don't notice it. When the following normal beat occurs after a slight pause, it will then feel much stronger than usual. PVCs may feel frightening, especially if you don't know what you are experiencing, but they are common and not dangerous. In fact, many women with PVCs are never even aware of them. When this arrhythmia originates in the atria, it is called premature supraventricular (or atrial) contraction. If you experience something that feels like an arrhythmia, remember that most are not serious. Nevertheless, you should ask your doctor to check your symptoms to determine the cause, especially if you feel dizzy or light-headed.

Treatment Options

Never try to self-diagnose an arrhythmia. Be sure to consult your doctor if you feel an irregular heartbeat that worries you. If you *are* diagnosed as having an arrhythmia, however, you may be able to learn to manage it by altering dietary or lifestyle habits that act as triggers. Something as simple as reducing or eliminating caffeine and/or alcohol, quitting smoking, or changing a medication may be the solution. If the arrhythmia persists, you have several treatment options, depending on the cause and your symptoms, medical history, and lifestyle. Drugs such as digitalis, beta-blockers, and calcium channel blockers, alone or in combination with other medications, can be used to effectively stop or control many arrhythmias. Other options include catheterization and ablation to eliminate the problematic electrical pathway or implantation of a pacemaker or implantable cardioverter-defibrillator (ICD).

coronary artery disease

Coronary artery disease (CAD) is caused by thickening of the walls of the arteries that supply blood to the heart muscle; those arteries are called the coronary arteries because they surround the heart like a crown. Narrowing of the coronary arteries reduces the amount of oxygen-rich blood delivered to the heart itself. When the blood flow is limited, the heart receives inadequate oxygen and nutrients, resulting in chest pain during exertion or stress. When blood flow is blocked completely, the heart muscle is deprived of all oxygen (myocardial ischemia), resulting in a heart attack (myocardial infarction). If the attack is severe enough, the oxygen-deprived heart tissue will die.

Arterial blockages can be triggered by spasms in the muscle cells or by inherited abnormalities, but most are caused by **atherosclerosis,** the gradual buildup of fatty streaks that harden into plaque lining the arterial walls. As plaque accumulates, it obstructs the flow of blood, narrowing the artery. If the plaque breaks or cracks, the blood clot that forms over the break may completely block the artery, causing a heart attack.

Angina pectoris, pain that is brought on by exertion, is a common symptom of coronary artery disease. **The classic experience of angina is a feeling of steady pressure in the chest, shoulders, arm, or jaw, but as a woman, you also can feel angina as shortness of breath or fatigue.** If your coronary arteries cannot widen to provide enough oxygen to the heart during exercise or stress, you will experience what is called *stable angina.* This condition goes away when you rest or take nitroglycerin, because the need for more blood is reduced.

Unstable angina, however, does not resolve with rest, or the pain may become more frequent, last longer, or occur during sleep. This form of angina is usually caused by reduced blood flow to the heart muscle because the coronary arteries are either narrowed by atherosclerosis or

What Is a Heart Attack?

A heart attack occurs when the blood supply to part of the heart muscle itself—the myocardium—is severely reduced or stopped. The reduction or stoppage happens when one or more of the coronary arteries supplying blood to the heart muscle is blocked. This is usually caused when arterial plaque bursts, tears, or ruptures, creating a "snag" where a blood clot forms and blocks the artery. If the blood supply is cut off for more than a few minutes, muscle cells suffer permanent injury and die. This can cause death or disability, depending on how much heart muscle is damaged.

Sometimes a coronary artery temporarily contracts or goes into spasm. When this happens the artery narrows and blood flow to part of the heart muscle decreases or stops. A spasm can occur in normal-appearing blood vessels as well as in vessels partly blocked by atherosclerosis. A severe spasm can cause a heart attack.

partially blocked by a blood clot. Another form of unstable angina is *variant angina,* which is caused by spasms in a coronary artery and may help explain heart attacks in younger women with little or no atherosclerosis. This is a much more serious condition that can warn of an impending heart attack. **If you experience angina that lasts longer than a few minutes, call 9-1-1 immediately.**

Treatment Options

The treatments for coronary artery disease vary depending on your personal health situation and the severity of the disease. Options include:

- Reducing pain and other symptoms with medication

- Opening blocked arteries with angioplasty and stents, atherectomy, and laser ablation

- Providing a new route around blocked arteries with coronary artery bypass surgery

Medications such as nitrates, beta-blockers, and calcium channel blockers act to relieve the symptoms of coronary artery disease, but they do not "undo" the narrowing or blockages of arteries. Nitrates cause the arteries to widen so blood can flow more easily. Beta-blockers reduce your body's need for more oxygen by interrupting signals telling your heart to work harder during exertion, thereby slowing heart rate and reducing blood pressure. Calcium channel blockers also reduce blood pressure and slow heart rate by causing the smooth muscle in the arteries to relax, allowing the arteries to widen.

Percutaneous coronary intervention (PCI) allows a physician to open up narrowed arteries that are reducing blood flow by using an inflatable catheter, a stent, or other devices. In this procedure, commonly known as *angioplasty,* a catheter with a balloon tip is inserted through the arteries to reach the plaque causing the blockage. The balloon is carefully inflated, literally flattening the plaque and widening the artery. In some cases, a stent made of very fine mesh is placed in the artery to maintain the opening created by the balloon. *Atherectomy* is similar to angioplasty, but instead of using a balloon to widen arteries, the catheter is equipped with a tiny high-speed drill that removes the plaque from the artery.

Coronary artery bypass surgery (CABG, pronounced "cabbage") provides a new route around a clogged artery by grafting a healthy artery or vein taken from elsewhere in the body. This widely used procedure offers relief if the blockage in your coronary arteries is too extensive for angioplasty, particularly if you have blockage in the main trunk of the left coronary artery or all three coronary arteries. Your surgeon has several options and can perform multiple bypasses, depending on your condition and how many arteries are blocked. An artery may be detached from the chest wall and the open end attached to the coronary artery below the blocked area, or a long vein in your leg may be removed, with one end sewn above the blockage and the other end attached or "grafted" to the coronary artery below the blockage. Either way, blood can use this new path to flow freely to the heart muscle.

peripheral vascular disease

Peripheral arteries and veins (those distant from your heart) can also be damaged, narrowed, or blocked by blood clots and inflammation. Just as in the coronary arteries, plaque can build up in the peripheral arteries, slowing blood flow and causing oxygen deprivation in the cells. Called peripheral artery disease (PAD), this common type of peripheral vascular disease often involves painful cramping in the hips, thighs, and calves during exercise, when tissues need more oxygen. The pain usually goes away within a few minutes when you stop exercising. That pain is called intermittent claudication and, like angina, is a symptom of the underlying condition of slowed blood flow rather than of a disease itself.

To diagnose peripheral vascular disease, your doctor will assess your description of your symptoms and measure the pulse in the arteries of your legs and feet. The **ankle-brachial index (ABI) test** compares the blood pressure in your feet to the blood pressure in your arms to determine how well your blood is flowing. Normally, the ankle pressure is at least 90 percent of the arm pressure, but with severe narrowing it may be less than 50 percent. Sonography, angiography, and arteriography also may be used to confirm the diagnosis.

The same factors that increase risk for coronary artery disease increase risk for peripheral vascular disease. **Smoking, high blood pressure, and diabetes are all major risk factors, so it's important to choose healthy lifestyle habits to protect your circulatory system.**

Treatment Options

Treatment of peripheral vascular disease focuses on reducing symptoms and preventing further progression of the disease. In most cases, lifestyle changes, exercise, and medications are enough to slow the progression or even reverse the symptoms of peripheral vascular disease. Unfortunately, this condition often goes undiagnosed, leading to painful symptoms or even loss of a leg. Peripheral vascular disease also increases your risk for heart attack and stroke, so be sure to discuss any symptoms you experience with your healthcare professionals.

heart failure

Although the name sounds frightening, the term "heart failure" does not mean the heart stops beating. Rather, it indicates a condition in which the heart keeps working but isn't efficient enough to pump an adequate supply of blood through the body. The sources of stress on the heart that can contribute to heart failure include high blood pressure, coronary artery disease, disease of the heart muscle (cardiomyopathy), disease of the heart valves, and infection of the heart valves and/or heart muscle (endocarditis and/or myocarditis), as well as scar tissue left from a past heart attack or congenital heart defects.

Cardiomyopathy is disease or infection of the heart muscle itself, often of unknown cause. Because this condition alters the muscle tone, the heart cannot pump as efficiently. Cardiomyopathy is relatively rare, but it is significant because it can cause sudden death if left untreated. Pregnancy may trigger cardiomyopathy in some women, even when no viral or bacterial infection is present. Why this happens is not known, although a genetic link is suspected. African American women in particular are at higher risk, as are women who are pregnant with twins. If you have a family history of cardiomyopathy and are thinking of becoming pregnant, it is important that you talk with your doctor about your risk for this disease and how to best manage your pregnancy.

With heart failure, in order to maintain blood flow, the failing heart will pump more often and the heart chambers will enlarge. At the same time, the kidneys will increase blood volume by retaining sodium and fluids. However, as blood flow out of the heart is reduced, blood returning to the heart through the veins backs up, causing congestion in the tissues. If more fluid accumulates than the kidneys can dispose of, the strain can compromise kidney function. Sometimes fluid also collects in the lungs and interferes with breathing, causing shortness of breath, especially when lying down. This condition is known as **congestive heart failure.**

The most common symptoms of heart failure are shortness of breath; fatigue; coughing, especially at night; swelling in the ankles, legs, and other parts of the body; and a need to urinate frequently at night. Because these symptoms can result from many causes, it's important for your physician to be able to consider them together in the context of your total heart health picture—another example of why you should communicate as much and as honestly as you can with your doctor.

Treatment Options

Depending on the cause, heart failure can be treated to alleviate symptoms in many cases. Lifestyle changes, especially restricting the amount of dietary sodium, and medications can reduce strain on the heart. Common drug therapies include diuretics, digitalis, vasodilators, and calcium channel blockers, which act to help reduce blood pressure, strengthen the heart, or allow blood to move more freely. In some cases, surgery can correct heart defects that lead to heart failure. If you have long-term heart failure that can't be treated by any other medical or surgical means, you may be a candidate for a heart transplant.

Because heart failure typically occurs *after* other heart-related conditions have developed, **it often is possible to avoid heart failure by choosing heart-healthy habits early on.** Identifying and managing risk factors such as high blood pressure, treating existing coronary artery disease, and correcting heart defects *before* heart failure develops are the best overall strategies.

disorders of the heart valves

As described in Chapter 2, the valves in your heart control the direction of blood as it moves from one chamber to the next. Their main function is to open and close in sequence as blood flows through the tricuspid valve to the right ventricle, then through the pulmonary (pulmonic) valve to the lungs. After the blood is oxygenated in the lungs, it flows through the left atrium, through the mitral valve to the left ventricle, and then through the aortic valve into the aorta. From the aorta it travels through the general circulatory system to deliver oxygen and nutrients to the body. At each stage of this delicate balancing act, the respective valves allow a certain amount of blood through and then snap shut. The resulting "lub dub" sound is what you hear through a stethoscope. If a valve problem exists, your doctor will hear a specific murmur in addition to the normal heart sounds and may order an echocardiogram to confirm the diagnosis.

When a valve does not close properly, blood can leak backward through the valve (called regurgitation or insufficiency). This reduces the volume of blood that travels through the cardiovascular system, so the heart must work harder to pump enough blood to the body. If a valve does not open properly (stenosis, or narrowing), it will restrict the flow of blood, also making the heart work harder to pump enough blood through it. Most valve disorders are not serious, but in some cases, if the problem is not corrected, over time the heart may gradually enlarge in response and become weaker and less efficient.

Typical Valve Problems and Treatment Options

Mitral valve prolapse (MVP) is the most common valve disorder, especially in women. With mitral valve prolapse, the leaflets, or flaps, of the mitral valve are enlarged and balloon out instead of closing properly. The cause is usually unknown, although some cases are hereditary. Most people with mitral valve prolapse don't have symptoms of the condition. More likely, your doctor will identify a click and/or a murmuring sound during a routine checkup. If you are told you have mitral valve prolapse, remember that generally the condition is benign and doesn't interfere with a normal, active life.

Backward blood flow from the left ventricle into the left atrium is called mitral regurgitation. Over time, this leakage of blood causes pressure in the lungs, leading to shortness of breath. The treatment for these mitral valve disorders will depend on how much blood is moving through the valve and the severity of symptoms. In most cases, no therapy is needed. If the leak is significant, your doctor may recommend restricted exercise, medication, or valve repair or replacement.

Mitral stenosis is the narrowing of the mitral valve. When this happens, the valve does not open enough to allow adequate blood flow. Although this condition can occur as a birth defect in rare cases, it usually develops as a result of rheumatic fever, which can damage the heart valves. Better prevention of rheumatic fever has made the condition much less common in developed countries these days, but once the stenosis is present, it can take years to identify the problem. The major symptom is shortness of breath because the narrowed valve increases pressure in the left atrium, causing congestion in the lungs. People with mitral stenosis can be treated with diuretics to relieve fluid congestion or surgery to repair or replace the valve.

Aortic regurgitation is a condition in which the aortic valve does not close completely and allows blood to flow back into the left ventricle. This disorder can result from untreated chronic high blood pressure, congenital heart disease, diseases such as infective endocarditis, Marfan syndrome, rheumatic fever, or calcium deposits on the valve leaflets (which occur with age). As with other valve defects, symptoms of this condition are typically not evident for years. If you have aortic regurgitation but do not experience symptoms, your doctor may prescribe medications to delay the need for further treatment. Because the left ventricle must work harder to compensate for the backward flow of blood, it can increase in size over time. Fluid also builds up, causing shortness of breath, chest pain, swelling in the ankles, and possibly even heart failure. If these symptoms become severe, your doctor may suggest valve replacement.

In the past, it was recommended that people with valve disorders take preventive antibiotics before certain dental, gastrointestinal, and gastro-urinary procedures to protect against infective endocarditis. Recently, the American Heart Association's Endocarditis Committee, together with national and international experts on endocarditis, extensively reviewed published studies and concluded that there is no conclusive evidence linking these procedures with the development of endocarditis. They also concluded that endocarditis is much more likely to result from frequent exposure to the random bacteria associated with daily activities. Therefore, the practice of giving patients antibiotics before a dental procedure is no longer recommended except for patients for whom endocarditis poses the highest risk.

Aortic stenosis is a narrowed opening of the aortic valve. It can be caused by congenital heart disease, rheumatic fever, or the buildup of calcium on the leaflets that can occur with age. All of these can reduce the blood flow from the left ventricle into the aorta. Again, the left ventricle must work harder to send the blood on to the rest of the body.

Aortic stenosis can lead to shortness of breath and dizziness. Exertion also might cause chest pain or palpitations. With severe aortic stenosis, blood flow to the brain may become dangerously reduced, resulting in fainting. If you have this condition, it is important to follow up with your healthcare provider anytime you experience increased shortness of breath or chest pain with exertion, since these symptoms require further investigation.

If the valve becomes very narrow, severe pressure builds up in the left ventricle, which can cause the heart to enlarge and weaken. When this occurs, it may be possible to enlarge the valve opening with a procedure called a balloon valvuloplasty. This technique does not repair the valve itself but will help reduce the narrowing and the pressure in the left ventricle. If the aortic valve begins to leak again over time after the procedure, however, it will probably need to be replaced.

congenital heart defects

Congenital heart defects are structural problems that occur when the heart or major blood vessels do not develop normally before birth. Most heart defects either cause blood to flow through the heart in an abnormal pattern or obstruct blood flow in the heart or vessels near it. Congenital defects range from a tiny pinhole between the heart's chambers—which either resolves or poses no threat—to serious malformations that can lead to congestive heart failure and other forms of heart disease. At least fifteen types of these defects have been recognized, with many individual variations. In most cases, doctors cannot determine the exact causes of these congenital problems. Genetic and environmental factors certainly have an impact, as do certain viral diseases or alcohol or drug abuse during pregnancy, but no one factor will necessarily lead to a heart defect.

As a fetus develops, it depends on its mother's circulatory system and placenta for oxygen and nutrients, so its blood flow through the heart is different before birth. In the fetal heart, the left pulmonary artery is connected to the aorta through a vessel called the ductus arteriosus, and the left and right atria are connected through an opening between them called the foramen ovale. Both of these conduits allow blood to bypass the baby's lungs as long as the baby is in the uterus and the baby's blood is oxygenated from the placenta. In most cases these pathways close up on their own once the baby is born. In some cases, however, these openings do not close when they should.

Sometimes there is an abnormal hole in the septum (the wall that separates the left and right atria and ventricles). These holes allow blood to leak backward in the wrong direction. A common congenital abnormality, **ventricular septal defect,** is a hole between the right and left ventricles. When there is a large opening between the ventricles, a significant amount of the oxygenated blood from the heart's left side is forced back into the right side, where it is again pumped to the lungs following the usual pathway. The extra blood being pumped into the lung arteries makes both the heart and lungs work harder, and the lungs can become congested. Over time, the heart may enlarge from the added work, and high blood pressure may occur in the lungs' blood vessels because of the increased volume of blood. If that happens, the blood vessel walls can be permanently damaged. On the other hand, if the opening between the ventricles is small, there is no strain on the heart and the only abnormal finding is a loud murmur. An **atrial septal defect** is an abnormal opening in the septum dividing the right from the left atrium. When the foramen ovale (the opening between the atria that is present in all babies when they are born but normally closes shortly after birth) fails to close, the condition is called **patent foramen ovale.** In the same way, the fetal opening between the aorta and pulmonary artery can fail to close, which is called **patent ductus arteriosus.** Other defects include tetralogy of Fallot, stenosis or narrowing in the aortic or pulmonary valves, transposition of the great arteries, coarctation of the aorta, atresia, and hypoplastic left heart syndrome. (For more detailed information on these and other heart defects, visit the American Heart Association Web site at www.americanheart.org.)

Even though most major defects are identified at birth, it's not uncommon for the more minor defects to go unnoticed until adulthood. Either during a routine heart examination or because symptoms appear, your doctor may discover that you have been living with some kind of congenital defect for years. For example, patent foramen ovale, often referred to simply as PFO, is present in about one in four women, yet most women have no symptoms and don't even know the defect exists. If you are told you have PFO, be reassured that it rarely causes adverse effects and typically needs no treatment.

reproductive health and congenital heart defects

If you know you have a significant heart defect, discuss the best form of birth control with your gynecologist or cardiologist. With many forms of heart disease, you can still use most of the effective methods safely. However, if you have complex heart disease, high blood pressure, or cyanosis (poorly oxygenated blood due to a heart defect), you should *not* use oral contraceptives because they increase the risk of blood clots. Intrauterine devices (IUDs) may predispose patients to endocarditis, an infection of the heart's inner lining or the heart valves. These devices generally are not recommended if you are at risk.

Many women with congenital heart defects can have a successful pregnancy, but it's wise to discuss your individual situation with your cardiologist before becoming pregnant. The physical changes of pregnancy, particularly in the second and third trimesters, can worsen the symptoms of congestive heart failure, or cause problems even if you've had no symptoms previously. With some types of heart defects, especially those associated with pulmonary hypertension or significant ventricular dysfunction, pregnancy creates significant risk for you. Your condition can also put the fetus at risk for poor growth or other problems. Several commonly prescribed heart disease medications pose added risks to the fetus. In many cases, you will be advised to have your pregnancy monitored by a high-risk obstetrician, often along with a cardiologist familiar with your condition. In addition, the risk of heart disease in the fetus is higher if either parent has a congenital heart defect. In these cases, your doctor may recommend an ultrasound to check the fetus's heart for possible defects.

• • •

If you've been diagnosed with a heart-related condition, your doctor will recommend the lifestyle changes and treatment plan that are best for you. Be sure to ask enough questions so that you understand your personal health issues and how they will affect your life. As a partner in your health care, discuss your test results, your diagnosis, and the available treatment options fully with your healthcare provider.

LOOKING TOWARD THE FUTURE

Scientific research is an open-ended endeavor. Sometimes, finding answers can raise new questions. In essence, the more we find out, the more there is to learn. What we can say for certain, however, is that ongoing research will lead to important health changes for women in the future. Just as women in their 50s or 60s now are experiencing improved health care because of past medical research, women in their 20s and 30s will enjoy better heart health 20 years from now because of the work being done today.

In the last 30 years, we have seen a major transition in the research community regarding women and heart disease. There is a growing awareness that women are different from men in ways that haven't been fully understood. This means there is a critical need for research into areas that specifically affect women, and in particular, the gender differences in heart-health issues. As part of its commitment to women and to advancing sound science, the American Heart Association spent more than $13 million in 2007 alone on research focused exclusively on women and cardiovascular disease. These and future studies will yield important discoveries, and the practical applications of those discoveries will enable more women to live healthier lives, perhaps free of heart disease for good some day.

genetics and heart health

One of the most exciting directions of current research is the arena of genetics and genomics, which offers new possibilities for both prevention and treatment of disease. Genome-wide association studies, for example, are being promoted to help identify the genetic variations associated with observable traits (such as blood pressure or weight) or with the presence or absence of a disease or condition. Scientists hope that by combining clinical data with whole genome information, they will be able to see how genes contribute to basic biological processes that affect one's health, and perhaps be able to predict disease or individual response to treatment. Genetic testing may then make it possible to personalize medical care based on a person's unique genetic material.

A major application of this research is genetic-based pharmacology. We already know that drugs can be metabolized differently by individuals, yet most drug prescriptions are currently based on very general population guidelines. In the not-too-distant future, a physician may be able to use genetic tests to identify how to best manage an individual's health care. For example, in recent studies of the drug warfarin, an anticoagulant that affects the body's clotting response, researchers have been able to predict drug dose and response using gene composition. In practice, this means that doctors will be able to tailor drug choice and dosage to a specific patient's needs—and thereby minimize the potential risk of that drug. For controversial agents such as hormone therapy, genetic testing may help identify those women who could benefit from hormone therapy without it increasing their risk of cardiovascular disease.

gender-based research

Additional areas of inquiry have garnered major funding from both the American Heart Association and the National Institutes of Health because they have such an impact on so many women and there is a clearly marked gender disparity.

Heart Attacks in Younger Women

Statistics show that currently younger and middle-aged women who have a heart attack have poorer recoveries than their male counterparts, including higher mortality. Recent research has clarified a number of ways atherosclerosis affects women differently than men, both in how it is distributed throughout the cardiovascular system and how it affects cardiovascular function. However, many questions remain unanswered about the mechanisms that contribute to the higher death rate after heart attack among younger women. Gender-specific areas of research include:

- the mechanisms that trigger heart attacks in younger women

- heart attack symptoms in younger women and, especially, the response to those symptoms by the medical community and the women themselves

- the continuum of care provided throughout and after a heart attack

- how to integrate secondary prevention into the lifestyle of young women

Arrhythmias and Cardiac Arrest

Women are at higher risk than men for certain types of arrhythmias that can lead to sudden cardiac arrest, but it's not clear why. To reduce the number of women experiencing and dying from sudden cardiac arrest, research is focusing on how gender plays a role in these areas:

- The effect of shifting hormone levels on cell membranes and their role in arrhythmia

- Biological mechanisms at the cellular level that may protect against arrhythmia

- How women may respond differently than men to therapies and devices used to treat arrhythmia

- Genetic clues as to why certain women may have a greater susceptibility to arrhythmia

Heart Failure in Older Women

There is a growing population of older women living with heart failure—an important public health issue with both human and economic implications. This prevalence of heart failure can be due to ischemic heart disease and viral cardiomyopathy, but also other illnesses that are specifically relevant for women, such as cardiomyopathy related to pregnancy, valvular heart diseases, and heart problems such as diastolic dysfunction. (Although we know that diastolic dysfunction is more common in women than men, there is no consensus yet on how to treat it.) Research is ongoing to help define the pathophysiology of these conditions and to determine the best treatment approaches.

Scientists are looking into:

- Gender differences in the specific causes of systolic and diastolic dysfunction

- The progression of steps leading to cardiac failure in women, and ways to interrupt it

- New ways to target and improve systolic and diastolic function

- Lifestyle and behavior changes that will help prevent heart failure as well as increase the effectiveness of therapy

our continued commitment

In addition to the research into these important topics, new advances will continue to improve the understanding of how being female affects heart health. Of course, no one study can provide definitive answers. The scientific process involves a lengthy progression of research and integration to build a useful knowledge base, particularly the type of knowledge that leads to safe prevention and treatment of disease in humans. As part of that process, the American Heart Association will continue to commit resources to the study of women's heart health and in turn translate the findings into practical and effective health care for women.

part four

resources

HEALTH SCREENING
BY DECADE

S tarting in your early 20s, you should get in the habit of scheduling regular health checkups—and you should strive to keep this habit throughout the course of your life. Regular checkups allow your healthcare providers to track changes in your health over time. Starting with a baseline measurement will give you and your future doctors a groundwork for comparison if your test numbers begin to change.

You can reduce the risk for heart disease if you start early. These important screening tests should be part of your ongoing medical checklist. On the following page, you'll find a quick-reference chart to help you keep track of what health screenings you'll need to get in every decade. But first, here's a quick snapshot of what to aim for as a result of the heart-related tests and screenings.

- **Body mass index (BMI):** Aim for between 18.5 and 24

- **Waist circumference:** Aim for less than 35 inches

- **Blood pressure:** Aim for less than 120 (mmHg) systolic and less than 80 (mmHg) diastolic

- **Lipid profile/cholesterol levels:** Aim for total cholesterol less than 200 mg/dL; LDL cholesterol less than 100 mg/dL if you have heart disease or diabetes; HDL cholesterol of 50 mg/dL or higher; triglycerides less than 150 mg/dL

- **Fasting blood glucose:** Aim for less than 100 mg/dL

HEALTH SCREENING CHECKLIST

	20s	30s	40s	50s	60s	70s+
Weight and BMI (every year)	✓	✓	✓	✓	✓	✓
Waist Circumference (every year)	✓	✓	✓	✓	✓	✓
Blood Pressure (every office visit or at least every 2 years, more often if at risk)	✓	✓	✓	✓	✓	✓
Lipid Profile/Cholesterol Levels (every 5 years, every year if at risk)	✓	✓	✓	✓	✓	✓
Heart Exam, including checking heart rate, pulse, breath sounds, heart sounds, skin color, and limbs for swelling (every 5 years, every year if at risk)	✓	✓	✓	✓	✓	✓
Eye Exam (every 2 years, *every 2 years if you have vision problems or at risk including diabetes or hypertension)	*	*	✓	✓	✓	✓
Glaucoma Test			✓	✓	✓	✓
Gynecological Exam, including breast and pelvic exams and a Pap smear (every year)	✓	✓	✓	✓	✓	✓
Mammogram (every year)			✓	✓	✓	✓
Fasting Blood Glucose (baseline by 45, every 3 years, *more often if you're pregnant, overweight, diabetic or at risk for diabetes, or if you have a history of gestational diabetes or polycystic ovary syndrome)	*	*	✓	✓	✓	✓
Colon Cancer Screening (every year with stool blood test, every 5 years with sigmoidoscopy, every 10 years with colonoscopy)				✓	✓	✓
Bone Density Scan (check when and how often with your doctor)				✓	✓	✓

HOW TO TALK
WITH YOUR DOCTORS

For the most effective health care, you need to work in partnership with doctors you trust. You expect your doctors to be knowledgeable and competent and to provide appropriate advice and treatment. You also expect the healthcare system to provide quality medical care. However, you need to be an active partner and play an important part in the process. Doctors do not always bring up heart disease with their female patients, especially with younger women, so it may be up to you to initiate the discussion. **The more you know about your heart and participate in your health care, the more you increase your chances of preventing or delaying heart disease and of receiving diagnoses and treatment when needed.**

establish a good relationship with your doctor

Make it a priority to work with a primary-care physician who fosters open communication—in both directions. Your doctor will ask you questions and should also listen carefully to your answers. Likewise, the more concrete information you can provide about your health and lifestyle, the more accurately your doctor can assess your situation and plan preventive care or identify a problem. Your honesty is important, since misinformation can lead to misdiagnosis.

listen to your body and tell your doctor about your symptoms

You intuitively know what's normal for you—and what's not. Even a general sense of "not feeling right" can be the tip-off to a serious condition, so **don't put off calling your doctor if that feeling persists.** If you wait for the feeling to go away by itself, you may be waiting for a heart attack instead. When you experience unexplained symptoms, write them down, as well as anything else you feel may be relevant, and note when the symptoms started and whether you have experienced them before. Take this information with you when you see your doctor. Don't feel embarrassed or afraid that your concerns will seem trivial. Listening to your body and communicating what you are experiencing to your doctor are essential components of both good preventive care and an accurate diagnosis.

Symptom Checklist

CHEST PAIN

- Is it constant or does it come and go? (If constant, get help immediately.)

- Is it localized or generalized; does it spread to your arms, shoulders, back, neck, or jaw?

- Is the pain mild, moderate, or severe?

- Does it feel dull, achy, or burning?

- How long does it last, and does it start suddenly or come on gradually?

- What triggers it—activity, stress, change in temperature?

- What relieves it—rest, warmth, movement such as walking?

- What other symptoms occur—nausea, vomiting, shortness of breath, dizziness?

SHORTNESS OF BREATH

- What triggers it—activity, stress?

- How long does it last?

- Does rest relieve it? Does lying down make it worse?

- Does it occur when you're asleep or lying flat on your back?

FATIGUE

- Have you had to stop normal activities because you feel drained of energy?

- Has it slowly gotten worse?

- Is it worse at the end of the day?

CHANGES IN HEART RHYTHM

- Do you feel your heart pounding, racing, skipping, or fluttering?

- What other symptoms occur—sweating, faintness, chest pain, dizziness?

LEG PAIN

- Is it localized or does it spread?

- Where is it—foot, calf, thigh, or buttocks?

- Does it feel like a cramp, or is it numbness, burning, or tingling?

- Does it occur with walking or at night while resting?

FAINTING OR DIZZINESS

- If you have fainted, was it after physical activity?

ABDOMINAL PAIN OR PRESSURE

- Where is the pain, and what triggers it?

schedule regular annual checkups and know your numbers

Routine exams will alert you and your doctor to developing health issues and risk factors so you can take preventive action. (See Appendix A for a health screening checklist by decade.) **Keep records of your test results** in case you need to change doctors or see a specialist.

ask questions and be proactive

After you share information about your heart health, it's your turn to **ask questions and to expect clear answers** that satisfy you. Even the best doctor can't know everything and won't have an answer for every question. However, if you feel that your symptoms are being dismissed or you need reassurance about a diagnosis, keep asking questions. If you feel your concerns are still not being addressed, consider seeing another professional for a different perspective. Don't be afraid that your doctor will be insulted. Most physicians welcome the opportunity to confer with their peers.

Be Prepared to Share

- Family and medical histories

- Current lifestyle habits, including typical eating habits, level of physical activity, smoking and drinking frequency, and sleeping patterns

- Recent changes in your usual routine

- Other factors that may be affecting your health, such as stress or emotional problems

What You Should Know

- Ask what your test results mean.

- If you are given a diagnosis, ask how the condition will affect you, and what options for treatment are appropriate.

- Discuss your lifestyle habits and ask about recommended changes in diet or physical activity. Ask for specific details if you are told to change your behavior, such as what foods or exercise routine would be best for you and what to avoid.

- If you are given a medication, ask when to take it and whether to take it with or without food, what to do if you miss a dose, when to expect results, what side effects to expect, and which foods or other drugs to avoid.

- After you begin a new medication, ask when you should return for a progress check to be sure the medication is working as it should. If it isn't, ask why.

- When you are given a medication by a specialist or any other healthcare provider, tell your primary doctor. Over-the-counter medications also can cause drug interactions with serious consequences, so ask your doctor or pharmacist about contraindications.

- If you need to manage risk factors such as high blood pressure and cholesterol, discuss the benefits and risks of each of the approaches your doctor has to choose from—before you start treatment.

- If you experience uncomfortable side effects from a medication, tell your doctor. Don't be stoic or stop taking the drug on your own. Every woman's body is unique, and your body's reaction to a certain drug is individual. You and your doctor may need to experiment until you find an option that works for you.

- If you are facing a decision about invasive diagnostic testing or treatment, ask what the desired goal is, what the options are, and what is involved in each alternative. Ask about side effects, how long you will need treatment, and whether you need to plan for recovery time.

- When you do schedule a test or procedure, ask how you will be given the results (for example, by mail or telephone) and who to contact in your healthcare provider's office if you have questions.

commit to your healthcare partnership

Studies show that **when you actively participate in your healthcare decision making, you are more likely to follow through with the lifestyle changes, diagnostic testing, and drug and treatment therapies your doctor recommends.** Having a comfortable working relationship with your doctors will increase your ability to identify developing heart disease in time to delay or prevent it, make educated treatment choices as needed, and enjoy the reassurance of being cared for by a professional you trust.

BASICS OF
HEALTHY WEIGHT LOSS

All successful strategies for effective and lasting weight loss depend on the same basic principle of balancing calorie intake with output of energy over time. A fad diet may cut back on calories but will not be sustainable, so chances are you will regain the weight you lose. Many women yo-yo from losing to gaining and back again, often putting on new pounds in the process. That's why the American Heart Association recommends that you **avoid fad diets and focus on finding an eating plan based on sound nutritional guidelines that you can follow for a lifetime.**

Calories In, Calories Out

It's a simple equation: **to lose weight, you need to take in fewer calories than you expend.** If you're not gaining weight or losing it, you're in "calorie balance," meaning that the amount of food you are eating is balanced by the energy you burn, regardless of how much you weigh at the time. To tip the balance toward weight loss, you need to determine your current calorie intake and dietary habits, then decide how you can subtract calories by reducing your intake and being more physically active.

In most cases, if you subtract 500 calories each day, you will lose about 1 pound per week, and if you subtract 1,000 calories a day, you will lose about 2 pounds per week. It's not a good idea to try to lose more than 2 pounds in one week without the supervision of a healthcare professional. Cutting back drastically to lose weight faster is generally not safe, and it can actually work against you if your body goes into starvation mode. That slows down your metabolic rate and your ability to burn calories.

Quality First, Then Quantity

As you subtract calories, you also need to **pay attention to the essentials of good nutrition.** Choose foods wisely so you can cut back on extra calories and transition to a healthful way of eating at the same time. **The key is making every calorie count.** To be sure you get all the nutrients your body needs, you should not eat less than an average of 1,200 calories daily except on the advice of a healthcare provider.

Move More, Weigh Less for Life

Although it's possible to initially lose weight by cutting calories alone, you need an exercise routine to keep off unwanted pounds. Healthcare professionals have found that **the best predictor of whether people will regain lost weight is whether they make physical activity a regular part of their lives.** If you want to maintain your weight loss for years, you must find ways to add more physical activity to your current lifestyle.

assess your current habits

Doing a self-assessment before beginning a weight-loss program will help you choose the approach that is most likely to work for you. What are your typical eating habits? Which of your food choices are most likely to lead to weight gain? What—if any—physical activity is part of your routine? What are the triggers that could overpower your best intentions?

Keep a diary for at least seven days (see the sample food diary template at the end of this appendix). Write down everything you eat and drink, and add up the calories for each item. Make a note of the time, as well as the reason, you ate what you did. Include any events that involve eating or drinking, from grazing at parties to finishing leftovers by the kitchen sink. Use the activity diary template (also at the end of this appendix) to record the minutes you spend being active, such as exercising at the gym, walking the dog, or doing energetic chores such as washing the car or preparing flower beds.

After a week of collecting data, add up all the calories you consumed during those seven days, then divide by 7 to find your daily calorie average. Do the same for your minutes of activity. As you review your diary entries, you'll also probably be able to identify harmful behavior patterns and repeated food choices that are high calorie but low in nutritional value—fast food, office munchies, and late-night TV snacks are common pitfalls. Decide how you can change the pattern or make substitutions to reduce total calories while maximizing nutritional payoff. Also look for the things you enjoy that you can make part of a healthy eating pattern, such as a favorite salad or restaurant choice. Identify the time of day when you feel most in control and when you tend to seek food for comfort or to relieve boredom. When are you most likely to be energetic and have time to add some exercise to your schedule? Use your observations to take advantage of your strengths and be aware of your weaknesses as you develop your weight-loss strategy.

calculate your calorie balance

In addition to the information from your diary, it's helpful to know how many calories you need to stay in calorie balance. Use the box on the next page to calculate the number of calories you can eat each day to maintain your current weight.

Compare your actual daily calorie average with the number you calculate from the formula in the box. The difference between the numbers will tell you whether you are in balance or are eating more than you need. If there is a large difference between the numbers, you will continue to gain weight, so you need to find ways to cut back.

Calorie Balance Worksheet

Multiply current weight in pounds _____ X 10 = **Base Calories** _____

Multiply current weight in pounds _____

If not active:	X 3	
If moderately active:	X 5	
If very active:	X 8 =	**Activity Calories** _____

Add Base + Activity Calories =
Total Calories to Maintain Weight _____

If you are older than 50 years, subtract 10% of that total.

(-10%) _____

Total Adjusted Calories _____

set your weight-loss goal

How much weight should you lose? Your primary goal is to achieve a heart-healthy weight without triggering a yo-yo pattern of loss and regain. **A good starting goal is losing about 10 percent of your current body weight.** For most women, a loss of between 10 and 20 pounds can bring noticeable health benefits.

Healthcare professionals use both body mass index (BMI) and waist circumference as indicators of overweight and obesity. To calculate your exact BMI, multiply your weight in pounds by 705. Divide by your height in inches; divide again by your height in inches.

- A BMI of less than 25 indicates that you are at a weight that is healthful for you (less than 18.5 is considered underweight, however).

- A BMI between 25 and 29.9 indicates that you are considered overweight.

- A BMI of 30 or more indicates obesity.

To use this chart to determine your BMI, find your height in the left-hand column and then move across to find your weight in pounds (pounds are rounded). The number at the top of the column is the BMI value for that height and weight.

BODY MASS INDEX (BMI)																	
	19	20	21	22	23	24	25	26	27	28	29	30	31	32	33	34	35
HEIGHT (INCHES)	BODY WEIGHT (POUNDS)																
58	91	96	100	105	110	115	119	124	129	134	138	143	148	153	158	162	167
59	94	99	104	109	114	119	124	128	133	138	143	148	153	158	163	168	173
60	97	102	107	112	118	123	128	133	138	143	148	153	158	163	168	174	179
61	100	106	111	116	122	127	132	137	143	148	153	158	164	169	174	180	185
62	104	109	115	120	126	131	136	142	147	153	158	164	169	175	180	186	191
63	107	113	118	124	130	135	141	146	152	158	163	169	175	180	186	191	197
64	110	116	122	128	134	140	145	151	157	163	169	174	180	186	192	197	204
65	114	120	126	132	138	144	150	156	162	168	174	180	186	192	198	204	210
66	118	124	130	136	142	148	155	161	167	173	179	186	192	198	204	210	216
67	121	127	134	140	146	153	159	166	172	178	185	191	198	204	211	217	223
68	125	131	138	144	151	158	164	171	177	184	190	197	203	210	216	223	230
69	128	135	142	149	155	162	169	176	182	189	196	203	209	216	223	230	236
70	132	139	146	153	160	167	174	181	188	195	202	209	216	222	229	236	243
71	136	143	150	157	165	172	179	186	193	200	208	215	222	229	236	243	250
72	140	147	154	162	169	177	184	191	199	206	213	221	228	235	242	250	258
74	148	155	163	171	179	186	194	202	210	218	225	233	241	249	256	264	272
75	152	160	168	176	184	192	200	208	216	224	232	240	248	256	264	272	279
76	156	164	172	180	189	197	205	213	221	230	238	246	254	263	271	279	287

Source: National Heart, Lung, and Blood Institute

Your waist circumference may tell even more than BMI about your risk for heart disease. Waist circumference is the distance around your natural waist, just above the navel. **If you have too much fat at your waist, you're at higher risk for health problems** such as high blood pressure, high blood cholesterol, and diabetes, which in turn increase your risk for heart disease. As a rule of thumb, aim for a waist circumference less than 35 inches.

american heart association
complete guide to women's heart health

choose a strategy to cut calories

To subtract between 500 calories and 1,000 calories from your current daily intake, choose a strategy that will suit your individual lifestyle. You can apply the following three core concepts to most real-life situations. You can also combine or swap approaches—whatever is most effective for you for the long term.

- **Substitute lower-calorie foods and beverages for high-calorie foods and beverages you consume on a regular basis.** Develop your calorie sense by reading calorie counters and food labels. Know the calorie count of every food you eat—before you eat it. You may be surprised by the high-calorie foods you eat often, and by the fact that there are lower-calorie options available. For example, a full-fat fruit yogurt can have up to 200 calories, while a fat-free plain yogurt with an added teaspoon of honey has only 100.

- **Reduce your overall intake by reducing the amounts of the foods and calorie-laden beverages you consume.** If you are in the habit of eating too much too often, this strategy may be the simplest way for you to start working toward a healthful weight. It's all about portion control: visualize what you would normally serve yourself, then eat only three-quarters of it. Part of ongoing weight control is learning what a reasonable portion should look like. For example, a 3-ounce portion of cooked meat is about the size of a computer mouse and one serving of pasta is about as big as a baseball.

- **Follow a formal meal plan that tracks both calories and nutrients,** such as the one described in the *American Heart Association No-Fad Diet* or as part of a commercial weight-loss program. If you prefer to have things spelled out with no guesswork, a defined-approach weight-loss program is a good option for you. You may find it easier to adhere to a healthy eating plan when you don't have to make many choices. As you follow an established program, you also will learn portion control and what foods are both low in calories and nutritionally sound.

All these approaches will help you cut calories, but they will have the most effect if you choose the ones that fit into your lifestyle and match your personal preferences.

make exercise a priority

It's true that calorie reduction is key to weight loss, but to keep the pounds off for good, you also need a regular routine of physical activity. Experts agree that **diet alone is not enough to keep you fit and trim over time.** In the same way you set your weight-loss goals, develop an exercise plan that will appeal to you through the decades and help protect your heart. If you're not active now, start by walking just an additional 10 minutes a day—as little as two 5-minute walks each day will start you moving. Once you're past the initial feeling of inertia, it will be easier to work up to the 30 to 60 minutes of daily exercise recommended for weight loss. If you are already moderately active, add to your current activities to reach an ideal goal of 60 to 90 minutes of exercise each day.

which activity is right for you?

Choose an exercise approach that fits your preferences and works with your usual routine. **When you enjoy an activity, you're more likely to stick with it.** Adding variety to your fitness plan so you'll have more fun also will help you keep motivated. Decide on a personal fitness goal and write it down. Then set aside a 30- to 60-minute block of time each day that you can devote to your plan without being interrupted. If finding time is difficult, schedule workout sessions on your calendar just as you would a dental appointment or a business meeting. When you give being active the same importance you give other aspects of your life, exercise won't slide to the bottom of your to-do list every day.

Here are some ways to get started:

- **Perform small activities throughout your day—on top of what you normally do—that add up to an increased amount of total activity.** Start at 10 minutes each day, and progress to 30 to 60 minutes each day. For example, find excuses to make extra trips up the stairs, whether climbing to your office instead of using the elevator or carrying laundry in three small batches instead of one large one. Rake leaves instead of using a leaf blower. The idea is to improve your physical fitness by finding ways to do more, not less.

- **Start a walking routine.** Walking is an ideal way to fit fitness into your life because it's inexpensive, easy, and convenient. Wear a reliable pedometer for one week to establish a baseline value for the number of steps you take daily. Then try to add about 250 steps each day. Between 5,000 and 7,000 steps is considered moderately active; 10,000 steps is very active. Each step counts toward your goal, so wear your pedometer as you walk your usual path around the grocery store, through the mall, or to a meeting. Include these measured segments of activity as part of your weekly routine until you are walking between 30 and 60 minutes a day.

- **Participate in scheduled classes such as yoga or aerobics or play organized team sports to increase your activity level.** Besides getting more fit, you'll benefit from the social support of your classmates and teammates. Find a friend who will join you and keep you going when you're tempted to skip a session.

Women of different weights burn calories at different rates, even when doing the same activity at the same intensity. In general, the heavier you are, the more calories you burn while doing a given activity. The chart on the next page will give you an idea of how many calories you use as you participate in various activities.

As you work toward your fitness goal, use simple checkpoints to measure your success. For example, how much less time did it take you today than last week to swim a lap or walk around the block? To stay on track, remember to monitor your progress and reassess every six weeks.

CALORIES BURNED IN 30 MINUTES OF CONTINUOUS ACTIVITY
(by approximate weight)

Activity	125 lbs	150 lbs	175 lbs	200 lbs	225 lbs
Badminton (social doubles)	113	135	158	180	203
Baseball and softball	118	141	165	188	212
Basketball	235	282	329	376	423
Bicycling	136	163	190	217	244
Bowling	82	98	114	130	147
Canoeing (at 2½ mph)	82	98	114	130	147
Cleaning windows	113	135	158	180	203
Gardening	163	195	228	260	293
Golfing (carrying the clubs)	128	165	193	220	248
Golfing (riding in a power cart)	82	98	114	130	147
Hiking and backpacking	170	204	238	272	306
Horseback riding (horse walking)	82	98	114	130	147
Horseshoe pitching	113	135	158	180	203
Ice and roller skating	163	195	228	260	293
Jogging (at 5 mph)	225	270	315	360	405
Jumping rope	313	375	438	500	563
Mowing (pushing a light power mower)	113	135	158	180	203
Mowing (riding lawn mower)	82	98	114	130	147
Racquetball	313	375	438	500	563
Raking leaves	128	165	193	170	248
Running (at 5½ mph)	264	317	370	422	475
Sailing (handling a small boat)	113	135	158	180	203
Sewing and knitting	57	68	79	90	102
Skiing (cross-country)	292	350	408	467	525
Skiing (light downhill)	188	225	263	300	338
Square dancing	188	225	263	300	338
Swimming	162	194	227	259	291
Tennis (singles)	197	234	271	310	349
Tennis (doubles)	138	165	193	170	248
Walking (strolling at 1 mph)	57	68	79	90	102
Walking (at 5 mph)	188	225	263	300	338
Water-skiing	188	225	263	300	338

Note: These figures are for comparison purposes only. Some of the activities are *not* aerobic exercise and burn very few calories.

stay motivated

It's exciting to get started on a new weight-loss program that you think will work for you. The hard part is maintaining that first burst of enthusiasm long enough to turn it into a lasting commitment. Try to remember that long-term success comes from progressive movement toward your goal. **Small changes on a daily basis really can bring big results.** Try these ideas to keep your motivation strong:

- **Keep your expectations realistic.** You didn't gain extra weight overnight, and you can't expect to lose it quickly either.

- **Anticipate plateaus.** An occasional slowdown of weight loss is normal. Stick to your plan and refocus when you hit a plateau. Think of it as a momentary stall, not a total breakdown. Try to find out what may no longer be working or may have changed. Look for new ways to cut back on calories or be more active.

- **Pay less attention to the numbers on the scale and more to how you feel in your clothes over time.**

- **Keep a written record of your progress** to help you focus better on your goals and remind you of your successes.

- **Try new combinations of eating plans and activity plans occasionally** to keep your choice tailored to your current needs.

- **Find a reliable source of support.** Family and friends can be helpful as you strive to maintain your weight-loss commitment.

- **Consider joining a weight-loss group or online program** with goals and approaches similar to yours.

- **Be prepared for life's inevitable crises.** If you now reach for food in times of stress, create an alternate plan so you will be ready to handle problems without relying on food.

With a positive attitude and a workable plan to tip your calorie balance in your favor, you can lose extra weight and keep from regaining it for the long term.

FOOD DIARY

DATE:_____ ☐ MON ☐ TUES ☐ WED ☐ THURS ☐ FRI ☐ SAT ☐ SUN

TIME/PLACE	FOOD OR BEVERAGE (TYPE AND AMOUNT)	CALORIES	WHAT PROMPTED YOU TO EAT?
BREAKFAST			
MORNING SNACK			
LUNCH			
AFTERNOON SNACK			
DINNER			
EVENING SNACK			

TOTAL DAILY CALORIES:_____

ACTIVITY DIARY

DATE:_____ ☐MON ☐TUES ☐WED ☐THURS ☐FRI ☐SAT ☐SUN

TIME OF DAY	ACTIVITY	DURATION	LEVEL OF EFFORT	LEVEL OF ENJOYMENT

TOTAL DAILY ACTIVITY MINUTES: _____

Notes:

IF YOU DID NOT EXERCISE TODAY, WHY?

☐ Not enough time

☐ Didn't want to

☐ Other

LEVEL OF PERCEIVED EFFORT

0 = Nothing at all
1 = Very, very light
2 = Very light
3 = Light
4 = Moderate/brisk
5 = Somewhat hard
6 = Hard
7 = Very hard
8 = Very, very hard
9 = Extremely hard
10 = Absolute maximal effort

ENJOYMENT

1 = Did not enjoy
2 = Neutral
3 = Did Enjoy

FAMILY HISTORY TREE

Like the color of your eyes, tendencies for many health conditions can be genetically passed on from one generation to the next. **If you have a blood relative with heart disease, your risk significantly increases.** The more you know about your family health history, the more you can do to protect yourself and reduce your risk of developing heart disease.

To get started, you'll need to identify your blood-related family members who have suffered a heart attack or stroke or who have lived with high blood pressure, diabetes, or other serious heart-related health conditions. Record this information on a copy of the tree diagram on the next page. Be sure to keep this document with your medical records and other important health information. Also, keep in mind that you'll want to update this diagram periodically.

Having a record of this information will be helpful not only to you now but also as you get older. Share this information with your doctor at your next visit. Talk to your healthcare provider about what your family history means for you and your heart health.

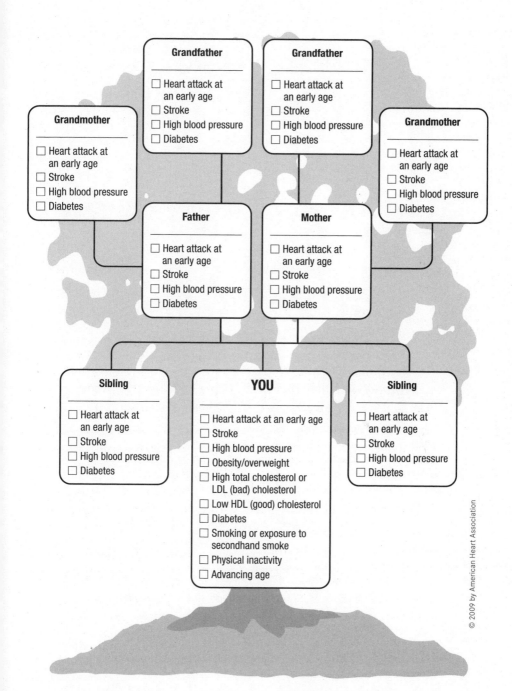

WARNING SIGNS OF HEART ATTACK AND STROKE

Know the Warning Signs of Heart Attack

If you have or see someone with any of the symptoms listed below, immediately call 9-1-1.

Warning Signs of Heart Attack

- **Chest discomfort.** Most heart attacks involve discomfort in the center of the chest that lasts more than a few minutes, or that goes away and comes back. The discomfort can feel like uncomfortable pressure, squeezing, fullness, or pain.

- **Discomfort in other areas of the upper body.** Symptoms can include pain or discomfort in one or both arms, the back, the neck, the jaw, or the stomach.

- **Shortness of breath.** This may occur with or without chest discomfort.

- **Other signs.** These may include breaking out in a cold sweat, nausea, or lightheadedness.

- As with men, women's most common heart attack symptom is chest pain or discomfort. But women are somewhat more likely than men to experience some of the other common symptoms, particularly shortness of breath, nausea/vomiting, and back or jaw pain. In addition, research suggests that indigestion and increasing fatigue may be experienced among some women having a heart attack.

Know the Warning Signs of Stroke

If you have or see someone with any of the symptoms listed below, immediately call 9-1-1.

Warning Signs of Stroke

- **Sudden numbness** or weakness of the face, arm, or leg, especially on one side of the body

- **Sudden confusion,** trouble speaking, or trouble understanding

- **Sudden trouble seeing** in one or both eyes

- **Sudden trouble walking,** dizziness, or loss of balance or coordination

- **Sudden, severe headache** with no known cause

AMERICAN HEART ASSOCIATION PROGRAMS AND RESOURCES

Go Red For Women

Go Red For Women is a national movement to bring awareness of heart disease to women by encouraging them to make good choices for their hearts and giving them tools to reduce heart disease. Learn more at GoRedForWomen.org.

Start!

Start! is a national call to action for all Americans and their employers to create a culture of encouraging physical activity and good health through walking so people will live longer, heart-healthier lives. To learn more, visit heart.org/start.

Power To End Stroke

Power To End Stroke is an education and awareness campaign that embraces and celebrates the culture, energy, creativity, and lifestyles of African Americans. The campaign calls on African Americans to help make an impact on the high incidence of stroke within their community. For more information, visit PowerToEndStroke.org.

The Heart of Diabetes

The Heart of Diabetes educates individuals about the connection between type 2 diabetes and cardiovascular disease. The campaign helps patients successfully manage their type 2 diabetes. For more information, visit IKnowDiabetes.org.

Search Your Heart

Search Your Heart is a nationally driven, community-based educational program whereby high-risk, diverse audiences receive training on three core topics to promote healthful lifestyles: heart disease and stroke, nutrition, and physical activity. For more information, visit americanheart.org/searchyourheart.

Heart Hub

Heart Hub is the American Heart Association's patient portal for information, tools, and resources on cardiovascular disease and stroke. Visit HeartHub.org for information on high blood pressure and details on managing your risks.

Cholesterol Web Site

The association's award-winning Web site americanheart.org/cholesterol helps the millions of Americans who have high cholesterol learn more about this major, but controllable, risk factor for heart disease.

Food Certification Program

The American Heart Association's heart-check mark helps you quickly and reliably find heart-healthy foods in the grocery store. When you see the heart-check mark on food packaging, you can have confidence knowing that the food has been certified by the association to meet our criteria for saturated fat and cholesterol. Visit heartcheckmark.org to learn more about how you can use the heart-check mark when you shop.

CPR Anytime

You can learn CPR in just 22 minutes at home. CPR Anytime and Infant CPR Anytime kits include reusable manikins in light-skinned or dark-skinned versions, instructional DVDs, and resource booklets to share with your entire family. For more information, visit cpranytime.org.

Consumer Publications

The American Heart Association offers a bestselling library of cookbooks and health books, including *American Heart Association Healthy Family Meals* and *American Heart Association No-Fad Diet.* Look for these and other American Heart Association books in traditional or online booksellers or visit americanheart.org/cookbooks.

GLOSSARY

ACE (angiotensin-converting enzyme) inhibitors—A class of drugs used to treat symptoms of heart failure and lower blood pressure while improving the pumping action of the heart. These agents work by interfering with the breakdown of angiotensin, a substance in the blood that causes vessels to tighten and raises blood pressure.

aerobic exercise—Brisk physical activity that requires the heart and lungs to work harder to meet the body's increased need for oxygen. Aerobic exercise promotes the circulation of oxygen through the cardiovascular system. Examples of aerobic exercise include running, swimming, and cycling.

alpha-blockers (alpha-adrenergic blockers or antagonists)—A class of drugs used to lower blood pressure and improve blood flow to the heart. These agents work to expand blood vessels and decrease resistance by lowering levels of angiotensin II. They allow blood to flow more easily and make the heart's work more efficient.

angina (angina pectoris)—Chest pain usually caused by inadequate blood flow to the heart muscle. Angina is a symptom of coronary artery disease that is usually experienced during activity and relieved by rest.

angiography—A diagnostic imaging technique used to examine the blood vessels and/or chambers of the heart. A dye visible by X-ray (contrast dye) is injected into the bloodstream and X-ray images are taken of its path through the cardiovascular system. The resulting images are called angiograms.

angioplasty—See *percutaneous coronary intervention (PCI)*.

angiotensin II receptor blockers—A class of drugs used to control blood pressure. Rather than lowering levels of angiotensin II as ACE inhibitors do, these agents prevent this chemical from having any effects on the heart and blood vessels, thus keeping blood pressure from rising.

angiotensin-converting enzyme inhibitors—See *ACE inhibitors*.

aorta—The major artery leading away from the heart. It receives blood from the heart's left ventricle and distributes it to the body.

aortic valve—The heart valve between the left ventricle and the aorta. It has three flaps, or cusps.

arrhythmia (dysrhythmia)—An irregular rhythm of the heart.

arteriography—A diagnostic imaging technique in which dye visible by X-ray is injected into the bloodstream. See *angiography*.

arteriole—A small, muscular blood vessel that branches from an artery and then extends to capillaries. Arterioles help regulate blood pressure by contracting and relaxing in response to various signals.

arteriosclerosis—A general term for thickening and hardening of the arteries.

artery—A large blood vessel that carries oxygen-rich blood away from the heart. The arteries branch into arterioles and then capillaries to transport the blood through the body. Arteries have thick, elastic walls that expand and contract in response to various signals to help regulate blood pressure.

atherosclerosis—A form of arteriosclerosis in which the inner layers of the artery walls become lined with fatty streaks that harden into plaque. As the plaque builds up, the arteries become narrow and less elastic, reducing the flow of blood.

atrium—Either one of the two upper chambers of the heart. The atria receive blood and move it to the ventricles, the two lower chambers of the heart. The right atrium receives oxygen-depleted blood returning from the body; the left atrium receives oxygen-rich blood returning from the lungs.

atypical symptoms—Symptoms of a heart attack other than chest pain. Women are somewhat more likely than men to experience atypical symptoms of a heart attack, particularly shortness of breath, nausea and vomiting, and back or jaw pain.

automated external defibrillator (AED)—An electronic device used to administer an electric shock through the chest wall to the heart. An AED helps reestablish the normal rhythm of contractions in a malfunctioning heart.

bacterial endocarditis—See *infective endocarditis*.

beta-blockers—A class of drugs used to treat high blood pressure, congestive heart failure, angina, and certain arrhythmias. Beta-blockers act to lower blood pressure by slowing the heart rate and decreasing the force of the heart's pumping action.

blood clot—A jellylike mass of blood tissue formed by clotting factors to stop the flow of blood from the site of an injury. Blood clots can form inside an artery whose walls are damaged by plaque buildup and can cause a heart attack or stroke by blocking blood flow.

blood pressure—The pressure of blood against the arterial walls. Blood pressure is measured when the heart contracts, called *systolic pressure*, and when the heart is at rest between beats, called *diastolic pressure*. Blood pressure is affected by the elasticity of the arterial walls and the volume of blood.

bradycardia—An abnormally slow heartbeat, defined as 60 beats or less per minute.

calcium channel blockers (calcium antagonists)—A class of drugs used to treat high blood pressure, arrhythmias, and angina. These agents block the movement of calcium into the heart and blood vessel muscle cells. This causes the muscles to relax, lowering blood pressure, slowing the heart rate, and lessening the heart's need for oxygen.

capillary—A microscopically small blood vessel branching from an arteriole. These blood vessels transport oxygen-rich blood to tissues throughout the body. The walls of capillaries are thin enough to allow the exchange of oxygen and nutrients for carbon dioxide and other waste products in the body's cells. Capillaries connect to veins for the blood's return to the heart and lungs.

cardiac arrest—The sudden cessation of the heartbeat, usually because of interference in signals from the heart's pacemaker. Cardiac arrest is usually associated with an underlying heart condition such as coronary heart disease or congestive heart failure.

cardiac catheterization—See *coronary angiography*.

cardiology—The study of the heart and its functions in health and disease.

cardiomyopathy—A serious condition affecting the heart muscle (myocardium). There are three types of cardiomyopathy: dilated, hypertrophic, and restrictive.

cardiopulmonary resuscitation (CPR)—A life-saving technique that consists of chest compression, sometimes combined with mouth-to-mouth breathing, to keep oxygenated blood flowing to the heart muscle and brain during cardiac arrest. CPR is used until an electric shock can be delivered to restart an adequate heartbeat or until advanced cardiac life support can be started.

cardiovascular system—The heart and its accompanying network of blood vessels. The blood vessels circulate blood from the heart throughout the body to supply tissue cells with oxygen.

cardiovascular—Pertaining to the heart and blood vessels. "Cardio" relates to the heart and "vascular" relates to the blood vessels.

carotid artery—The main artery in the neck. It supplies oxygenated blood to the brain. Blockages in this artery or its branches can cause a stroke.

cholesterol—A soft, waxy substance found among the lipids (fats) in the bloodstream and in the body's cells. Produced by the liver, cholesterol is used to form cell membranes and some hormones and is needed for other body functions. Because cholesterol cannot dissolve in blood, it must be transported to and from cells by carriers called lipoproteins. Three types of lipid make up the major part of the total blood cholesterol measurement: HDL cholesterol, LDL cholesterol, and triglycerides. Eating a diet rich in foods containing saturated fat, trans fat, and dietary cholesterol can lead to an excess of cholesterol in the bloodstream.

circulation—The movement of blood through the cardiovascular system.

computed tomography (CT or CAT scan)—A noninvasive imaging technology that uses computer analysis of X-ray imaging to produce cross-sectional images of the chest, including the heart and blood vessels. CT scans are more detailed than a standard X-ray.

congenital heart defect—A malformation of the heart or its major blood vessels that is present at birth.

congestive heart failure—A form of heart failure. Because the weakened heart is unable to effectively pump oxygenated blood out of the heart, the remaining blood backs up in the veins leading to the heart, causing congestion in body tissues and sometimes accumulation of fluid in the body, particularly the lungs and legs.

coronary angiography—A diagnostic imaging technique used to find narrowing or blockage in the coronary arteries. During the procedure, a catheter led by a guide wire is inserted into the femoral artery of the leg and slowly threaded up into the aorta. Once the catheter is in place, a dye visible by X-ray (contrast dye) is injected into the bloodstream through the catheter. Areas of narrowing can then be seen on a video screen and recorded. Blood samples can be taken and blood pressures measured through the catheter as well.

coronary arteries—Two main arteries that receive oxygenated blood from the aorta and branch off into a network of smaller arteries that feed blood directly to the heart muscle.

coronary artery bypass surgery (CABG or "cabbage")—A surgical procedure used to improve the blood supply to the heart muscle. One or more segments of healthy blood vessel are taken from another part of the body and grafted above and below the obstructed artery to allow blood to flow freely to the heart.

coronary artery disease (CAD)—A condition caused by narrowing of the coronary arteries so that blood flow to the heart muscle is reduced. The reduced supply of oxygen to the heart tissues causes chest pain called angina. The more the flow of blood providing oxygen is blocked, the greater the risk for heart attack (myocardial infarction).

cyanosis—A condition in which the skin appears bluish, especially the fingers, toes, and lips, because of poorly oxygenated blood. Cyanosis can result from congenital heart defects that cause blood to circulate abnormally.

defibrillator—See *automated external defibrillator*.

diabetes (diabetes mellitus)—A disease in which the body either doesn't produce enough of the hormone insulin or cannot metabolize it. Insulin is used to convert sugars into energy. When insulin is not metabolized efficiently, the resulting excess of glucose in the blood (also called blood sugar) causes damage if not controlled.

diastolic blood pressure—The pressure of blood against the arterial walls when the heart is at rest between beats.

digitalis—See *digoxin*.

digoxin—A drug used to treat moderate to severe heart failure and certain arrhythmias. Digoxin strengthens the contraction of the heart muscle and slows the heart rate.

diuretics—A class of drugs used to treat high blood pressure, heart failure, and some congenital heart defects. These agents cause the body to rid itself of excess fluids and sodium through urination. This helps reduce the heart's workload and decreases the buildup of fluid in the lungs and other parts of the body, such as ankles and legs. Different diuretics remove fluid at varied rates and through different methods.

Doppler ultrasound—A noninvasive imaging technology that uses ultrasound (high-frequency sound vibrations) to monitor blood flow, identify blood vessels that may be narrowing, and diagnose other vascular and heart conditions.

echocardiography—A noninvasive diagnostic technique that uses sound waves transmitted through the body to produce two- or three-dimensional images of the surfaces and movements of the heart and surrounding structures. A stress echocardiogram is recorded before and during, or immediately after, some form of physical stress, such as exercise on a stationary bicycle or treadmill.

edema—Swelling caused by an accumulation of fluid in body tissues. Edema in the legs, ankles, and lungs is common with heart failure.

electrocardiogram (ECG or EKG)—A graphic record of the heart's electrical impulse produced with electrocardiography.

electrocardiography—A noninvasive diagnostic technology that monitors the electrical activity associated with the heartbeat.

embolus—A blood clot that moves through the bloodstream until it lodges in a narrowed vessel and blocks blood flow.

estrogen replacement therapy (ERT)—See *hormone replacement therapy (HRT)*.

exercise stress test—A diagnostic test used to evaluate coronary blood flow in response to exercise, often used to diagnose coronary artery disease. During the test, a person walks on a treadmill or pedals a stationary bicycle while wearing electronic sensors that monitor the heart. Technicians monitor the person's heart rate, breathing, blood pressure, level of fatigue, and the electrical activity of the heart as recorded on an electrocardiogram.

fibrillation—Fast uncoordinated contractions of individual heart muscle fibers. A heart chamber in fibrillation cannot contract effectively and pumps blood inefficiently, if at all.

HDL cholesterol—The level of helpful or "good" cholesterol in the blood. See *high-density lipoprotein (HDL)*.

heart attack—A sudden obstruction of the blood flow through a coronary artery, causing damage to or death of heart tissue. See *myocardial infarction*.

heart failure—A condition in which the heart cannot pump enough oxygen-rich blood to meet the body's needs. Some of the symptoms are tiredness, shortness of breath, and swelling in the feet, ankles, and legs.

heart murmur—An abnormal sound heard in the heart as blood circulates through the heart's chambers, valves, or nearby blood vessels. Murmurs can result from defective heart valves or holes in the heart walls or be caused by pregnancy, fever, thyrotoxicosis (a condition resulting from an overactive thyroid gland), or anemia.

high blood pressure (hypertension)—A chronic elevation of arterial blood pressure above its normal range. Blood pressure that measures over 140 mmHg (systolic pressure) and 90 mmHg (diastolic pressure) on two or more separate occasions is classified as high.

high-density lipoprotein (HDL)—A cholesterol-carrying lipoprotein that may protect against heart disease by transporting cholesterol away from existing arterial plaque and removing it from the bloodstream.

hormone replacement therapy (HRT)—A therapeutic method of replacing the hormones estrogen and progesterone in women who have gone through menopause naturally or who have undergone a hysterectomy.

hypertension—See *high blood pressure.*

hypotension—Abnormally low blood pressure.

implantable cardioverter-defibrillator (ICD)—An electronic device inserted surgically to correct life-threatening heart rhythms.

infective endocarditis—A bacterial infection of the heart's inner lining (endocardium) or the heart valves that can damage or destroy the heart valves. Although endocarditis is rare in women with normal hearts, the risk is increased for women with damaged heart valves, artificial valves, congenital heart defects, or a history of previous endocarditis.

insulin resistance—A condition in which the body cannot metabolize insulin efficiently. As blood sugar levels rise, the pancreas works to release more insulin to compensate. The insulin-producing cells of the pancreas gradually become defective and decrease in number, allowing rising blood sugar levels to develop into full-blown diabetes.

ischemia—Decreased blood flow to the heart or brain, usually caused by narrowing or obstruction of an artery.

LDL cholesterol—The level of harmful or "bad" cholesterol in the blood. See *low-density lipoprotein (LDL).*

lipid profile—A fasting blood test that includes measurements of total cholesterol, HDL cholesterol, LDL cholesterol, and triglycerides.

lipid—A fatty substance such as cholesterol and triglyceride that is insoluble in blood.

lipoprotein—A particle complex composed of a lipid (fat) surrounded by a protein so that the lipid is soluble in blood. Lipoproteins are characterized by their density: high-density lipoprotein (HDL), low-density lipoprotein (LDL), and very low-density lipoprotein (VLDL). The lipoprotein particle carries all types of lipids, including cholesterol, through the bloodstream.

low-density lipoprotein (LDL)—A cholesterol-carrying lipoprotein that contributes to the buildup of plaque in blood vessels; plaque buildup is associated with coronary artery disease and other forms of heart disease.

magnetic resonance angiography (MRA)—A noninvasive imaging technology that uses magnetic resonance imaging and a contrast dye to identify obstructed blood vessels.

magnetic resonance imaging (MRI)—A noninvasive imaging technology that uses signals emitted from the body in response to a magnetic field. These signals are computer generated into detailed pictures of the heart and other structures without a dye being injected. MRI images can identify various heart problems, such as damage from a heart attack.

metabolic syndrome—A group of three or more metabolic risk factors that exist in one person, including overweight/obesity, insulin resistance, physical inactivity, lipid abnormalities, high blood pressure, and high fasting blood glucose.

metabolism—The set of chemical processes that maintain the cells in the body by breaking down and synthesizing sources of energy.

mitral valve prolapse—A condition in which one or both mitral valve flaps or leaflets balloon out instead of closing smoothly when the heart pumps, thus allowing blood to flow backward into the left atrium.

mitral valve—The heart valve between the left atrium and the left ventricle. It has two flaps, or cusps.

monounsaturated fat—A type of fat found in many foods, including vegetable oils such as olive, canola, peanut, sunflower, and sesame. Other sources include avocados, peanut butter, and many nuts and seeds. Monounsaturated fats are typically liquid at room temperature but start to turn solid when chilled.

myocardial infarction—A sudden obstruction of the blood flow through a coronary artery, causing death of part of the heart muscle (commonly referred to as heart attack). Myocardial infarction is diagnosed by clinical signs, electrocardiogram, and the presence of certain blood enzymes released from the damaged heart tissue.

myocarditis—An infection of the muscle tissue of the heart.

myocardium—The muscle tissue of the heart that rhythmically contracts and relaxes to pump blood through the heart.

nitroglycerin—A drug that is used to treat acute chest pain (angina). Nitroglycerin relaxes and dilates blood vessels, allowing an increased supply of blood and oxygen to the heart while reducing its workload. "Nitro" is prescribed as quick-dissolving pills to be placed under the tongue when needed.

obesity—The condition of being 30 percent or more over ideal body weight. Obesity strains the heart, increases the likelihood of high blood pressure and diabetes, and is a major risk factor for cardiovascular disease.

open-heart surgery—A surgical procedure performed on the opened heart while the bloodstream is diverted through a heart-lung machine.

pacemaker—A small battery-operated device inserted under the skin of the chest or abdomen to help manage abnormal heart rhythms. Pacemakers send electrical pulses to prompt the heart to beat at a normal rate.

palpitations—The sensation of the heart beating rapidly or irregularly.

percutaneous coronary intervention (PCI)—Commonly referred to as angioplasty, this invasive procedure is used to improve blood flow to the heart by dilating (opening) narrowed arteries. In most cases, a catheter with a deflated balloon on its tip is passed into the narrowed artery segment. The balloon then is carefully inflated, literally flattening the plaque and widening the artery. PCI may involve other procedures such as atherectomy or implanting stents.

pericarditis—Inflammation of the protective membrane surrounding the heart (pericardium), characterized by sharp pain behind the breastbone on the left side of the chest.

pericardium—A protective membrane that holds the heart and blood vessels in place while allowing the heart to move during its cycle of contractions.

peripheral artery disease (PAD)—A condition in which plaque builds up on the walls of the arteries leading to the kidneys, stomach, arms, legs, and feet. As occurs in coronary artery disease, the resulting blockages restrict blood circulation, causing cramping or fatigue in the legs and buttocks during activity. PAD is the most common type of peripheral vascular disease.

plaque (atheroma)—A raised deposit of fatty substances (including choles-terol, calcium, cellular waste, and others) that develops along the inner lining of arteries and small blood vessels. Plaque contributes to the nar-rowing and hardening of the arteries associated with atherosclerosis and arteriosclerosis.

polyunsaturated fat—A type of fat found mostly in grain products; vegetable oils such as soybean, corn, and safflower; and fatty fish such as salmon, mackerel, herring, and trout. Other sources include some nuts and seeds, such as walnuts and sunflower seeds. Polyunsaturated fats are typically liquid at room temperature and when chilled.

positron emission tomography (PET scan)—A noninvasive diagnostic tech-nique that uses positron-emitting substances to demonstrate whether heart muscle is alive and functioning properly.

prehypertension—A slightly elevated blood pressure approaching unhealthy levels. Prehypertension is defined as levels of systolic blood pressure between 120 and 139 mmHg and diastolic blood pressure between 80 and 89 mmHg.

premature atrial contraction—An early beat of the heart's upper chamber (atrium) that may feel like an irregular or skipped heartbeat.

premature ventricular contraction—An early beat of the heart's lower cham-ber (ventricle) that may feel like palpitations or an irregular or skipped heartbeat. The early beat often is not felt, and the next regular beat will feel stronger than usual, so it may seem as if the heart is pounding.

pulmonary valve—The heart valve between the right ventricle and the pulmo-nary artery. It has three flaps, or cusps.

rheumatic heart disease—A condition resulting from damage done to the heart, particularly the heart valves, by one or more attacks of rheumatic fever.

risk factor—A condition that is associated with an increased chance of devel-oping cardiovascular disease, including stroke.

saturated fat—A type of fat found mainly in foods from animal sources such as meat and dairy products. Saturated fats are typically solid at room temperature.

silent ischemia—Episodes of ischemia (decreased blood flow) that are not accompanied by pain.

sinoatrial node—A natural pacemaker composed of specialized heart muscle cells located in the right atrium. The sinoatrial node produces the electrical impulses that trigger the atria to contract at regular intervals. These impulses are produced at a steady rate, but external factors can affect the rate of discharge, allowing the heart to respond to varying demands. Also called *sinus node.*

sodium—A mineral that, together with potassium and calcium, regulates the body's water balance, maintains normal heart rhythm, and is responsible for nerve impulse conduction and muscle contraction. Excessive intake of sodium from food contributes to high blood pressure in some people.

statins—A class of drugs used to reduce blood levels of harmful LDL cholesterol, which is associated with increased risk of cardiovascular disease. These agents work in the liver to prevent the formation of cholesterol. Statins are most effective at lowering LDL cholesterol but also have modest effectiveness in lowering triglyceride levels and raising levels of helpful HDL cholesterol.

stenosis—The narrowing of an artery, valve, or other organ that results in slowing the flow of blood.

stent—A tiny wire mesh tube that is placed permanently in a narrowed artery to keep the artery open after angioplasty.

stress—Bodily or mental tension in response to physical, chemical, or emotional factors. Stress can refer to physical exertion as well as mental anxiety.

stroke—A sudden interruption of the blood flow to the brain that causes damage to or death of brain tissue. Stroke may be caused by a blockage in an artery that feeds the brain, a blood clot that obstructs a blood vessel in the brain, or bleeding in the brain. Stroke may cause temporary or permanent paralysis, slurred speech, and/or altered brain function.

systolic blood pressure—The pressure against the arterial walls when the heart contracts with each heartbeat.

tachycardia—An abnormally fast heartbeat, defined as greater than 100 beats per minute. Supraventricular tachycardia originates in the atria. Ventricular tachycardia originates in the ventricles.

thallium stress test—A diagnostic test used to detect coronary artery blockage and identify damaged heart muscle after a heart attack. During the test, a person walks on a treadmill or pedals a stationary bicycle. Thallium, a radioactive isotope, is injected into a vein during exercise, and an X-ray scanner is used to follow the path of the thallium as it is carried by the blood into the heart muscle.

thrombosis—The formation or presence of a blood clot (thrombus) inside a blood vessel or in a heart cavity. A clot that forms in the arterial system, called arterial or coronary thrombosis, can cause a heart attack or stroke.

trans fat (trans fatty acids)—A type of fat created in the industrial process that adds hydrogen to liquid vegetable oils to make them more solid (hydrogenation). Trans fats raise harmful LDL cholesterol levels and lower helpful HDL cholesterol levels. Trans fats can be found in many fried foods, baked goods, and stick margarines, and are listed as "partially hydrogenated oils."

transesophageal echocardiography (TEE)—A diagnostic technique that uses an ultrasound transducer introduced into the esophagus to produce three-dimensional images of the heart and its movements. Because TEE images provide very clear pictures of the heart's valves and chambers without the obstruction of the ribs or lungs, this test is used when the results from a standard echocardiogram are not sufficient.

transient ischemic attack (TIA)—A strokelike event that is caused by a temporarily blocked blood vessel and lasts only a short time.

treadmill test—See *exercise stress test*.

tricuspid valve—The heart valve between the right atrium and right ventricle. It has three flaps, or cusps.

triglyceride—The chemical form of most fats existing in food or in the body. Triglycerides present in the bloodstream are derived from fats eaten in foods or made in the body from other energy sources, such as carbohydrates. Calories eaten in a meal and not used immediately by tissues are converted to triglycerides and transported to fat cells to be stored.

vascular—Pertaining to blood vessels.

vein—A blood vessel that carries blood from the capillaries in the body's tissues back to the heart.

ventricle—Either one of the two lower chambers of the heart. The ventricles receive blood from the atria, the two upper chambers of the heart. The right ventricle pumps oxygen-depleted blood to the lungs. The left ventricle pumps oxygen-rich blood to tissues throughout the body.

ventricular fibrillation—A lethal irregular heartbeat in which the heart's electrical activity becomes disordered and the heart begins to beat very rapidly, reaching up to 300 beats per minute. This serious condition requires immediate medical help, beginning with cardiopulmonary resuscitation. Shocking the heart with an automated external defibrillator may restart a regular heartbeat.

venule—A tiny vessel that collects blood from the capillary beds and feeds into the veins.

very-low-density lipoprotein (VLDL)—A cholesterol-carrying lipoprotein that also transports triglycerides through the bloodstream.

INDEX